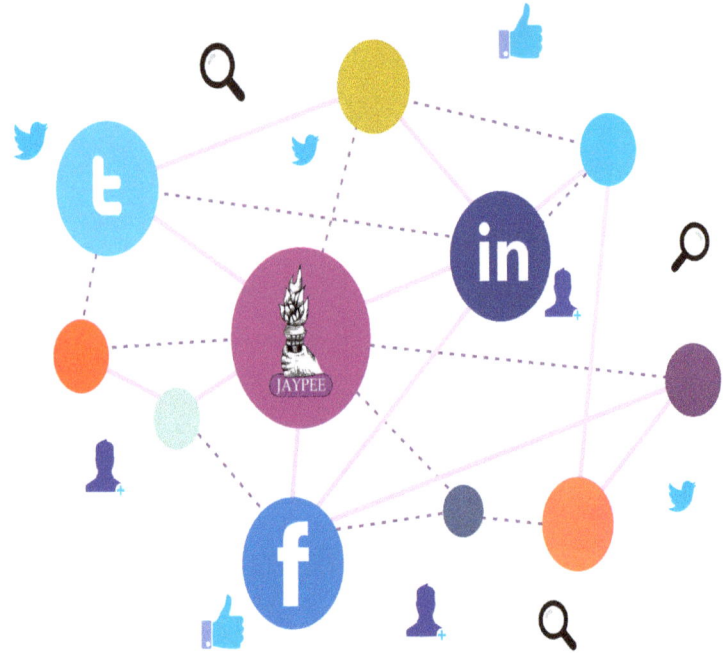

## Follow | Like | Explore

Join India's Premier Health Sciences Publisher JAYPEE

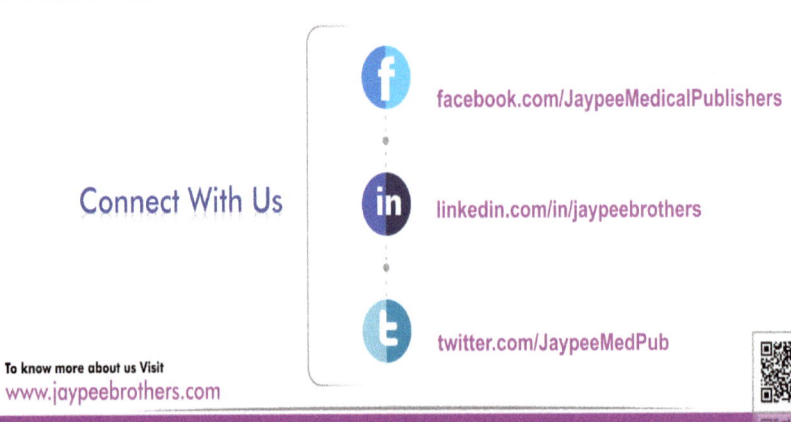

# Handbook of
# TRANSURETHRAL RESECTION (TUR) TECHNIQUE

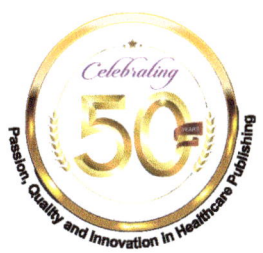

# Handbook of
# TRANSURETHRAL RESECTION (TUR) TECHNIQUE

*Editor*

**M Anandan**
MS MCh Fellowship in Minimally Invasive Urology (Robotic Surgery)
Consultant Urologist
Kovai Medical Center and Hospital
Coimbatore, Tamil Nadu, India

*Foreword*

**PN Dogra**

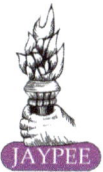

**JAYPEE BROTHERS MEDICAL PUBLISHERS**
*The Health Sciences Publisher*
New Delhi | London | Panama

**Jaypee Brothers Medical Publishers (P) Ltd.**

**Headquarters**
Jaypee Brothers Medical Publishers (P) Ltd
4838/24, Ansari Road, Daryaganj
New Delhi 110 002, India
Phone: +91-11-43574357
Fax: +91-11-43574314
E-mail: jaypee@jaypeebrothers.com

**Overseas Offices**

J.P. Medical Ltd
83, Victoria Street, London
SW1H 0HW (UK)
Phone: +44 20 3170 8910
Fax: +44 (0)20 3008 6180
E-mail: info@jpmedpub.com

Jaypee-Highlights Medical Publishers Inc
City of Knowledge, Bld. 235, 2nd Floor, Clayton
Panama City, Panama
Phone: +1 507-301-0496
Fax: +1 507-301-0499
E-mail: cservice@jphmedical.com

Jaypee Brothers Medical Publishers (P) Ltd
Bhotahity, Kathmandu, Nepal
Phone: +977-9741283608
E-mail: kathmandu@jaypeebrothers.com

Website: www.jaypeebrothers.com
Website: www.jaypeedigital.com

© 2019, Jaypee Brothers Medical Publishers

The views and opinions expressed in this book are solely those of the original contributor(s)/author(s) and do not necessarily represent those of editor(s) of the book.

All rights reserved. No part of this publication may be reproduced, stored or transmitted in any form or by any means, electronic, mechanical, photocopying, recording or otherwise, without the prior permission in writing of the publishers.

All brand names and product names used in this book are trade names, service marks, trademarks or registered trademarks of their respective owners. The publisher is not associated with any product or vendor mentioned in this book.

Medical knowledge and practice change constantly. This book is designed to provide accurate, authoritative information about the subject matter in question. However, readers are advised to check the most current information available on procedures included and check information from the manufacturer of each product to be administered, to verify the recommended dose, formula, method and duration of administration, adverse effects and contraindications. It is the responsibility of the practitioner to take all appropriate safety precautions. Neither the publisher nor the author(s)/editor(s) assume any liability for any injury and/or damage to persons or property arising from or related to use of material in this book.

This book is sold on the understanding that the publisher is not engaged in providing professional medical services. If such advice or services are required, the services of a competent medical professional should be sought.

Every effort has been made where necessary to contact holders of copyright to obtain permission to reproduce copyright material. If any have been inadvertently overlooked, the publisher will be pleased to make the necessary arrangements at the first opportunity. The **CD/DVD-ROM** (if any) provided in the sealed envelope with this book is complimentary and free of cost. **Not meant for sale.**

**Inquiries for bulk sales may be solicited at:** jaypee@jaypeebrothers.com

*Handbook of Transurethral Resection (TUR) Technique*

*First Edition:* **2019**

ISBN: 978-93-5270-398-2

**Dedicated to**

*My teachers and my family.*

# Contributors

**Arunkumar** MS MRCS DNB MCh
Consultant Urologist
RG Urology and Laparoscopic Hospital
Chennai, Tamil Nadu, India

**C Ramesh** MS MCh
Registrar Department of Urology
Kovai Medical Center and Hospitals
Coimbatore, Tamil Nadu, India

**Deepak Rathi** MS DNB
Senior Fellow
Medanta Kidney and Urology Institute
Medanta—The Medicity
Gurugram, Haryana, India

**Ganesh Gopalakrishnan** MS MCh
Consultant Urologist
Vedanayagam Hospital
Coimbatore, Tamil Nadu, India

**K Senthil** MS FRCS MCh
Consultant Urologist
Urology Clinic and Ganga Uro and
Nephro Center
Coimbatore, Tamil Nadu, India

**Mallikarjuna Chiruvella** MS MCh
Managing Director and
Senior Consultant Urologist
Asian Institute of Nephrology and Urology
Hyderabad, Telangana, India

**M Anandan** MS MCh Fellowship in Minimally Invasive Urology (Robotic Surgery)
Consultant Urologist
Kovai Medical Center and Hospital
Coimbatore, Tamil Nadu, India

**Md Taif Bendigeri** MS MCh
Consultant Urologist
Asian Institute of Nephrology and Urology
Hyderabad, Telangana, India

**N Selvarajan** MD
Senior Consultant and Head
Department of Anesthesiology
Kovai Medical Center and Hospital
Coimbatore, Tamil Nadu, India

**Narmada P Gupta** MS MCh FAMS DSc
Chairman, Academic and Research Urology
Medanta Kidney and Urology Institute
Medanta—The Medicity
Gurugram, Haryana, India

**PVLN Murthy** MS MCh
Senior Consultant Urologist
Kamineni Hospitals
Hyderabad, Telangana, India

**R Manikandan** MS MCh
Additional Professor
Department of Urology
JIPMER
Puducherry, Tamil Nadu, India

**RM Meyyappan** MS MCh
Professor and Head
Department of Urology
SRM Medical College Hospital and
Research Centre
Chennai, Tamil Nadu, India

**R VijayaWkumar** MS MCh MNAMS FRCS
Medical Director and Chief Urologist
RG Urology and Laparoscopic Hospital
Chennai, Tamil Nadu, India

# Foreword

I am delighted to introduce the *Handbook of Transurethral Resection (TUR) Technique* of the prostate and bladder tumor edited by M Anandan. I have known M Anandan as a resident fellow while his rotation in urology during his training in surgery at All India Institute of Medical Sciences (AIIMS), New Delhi, India. He is a very keen observer and academician at heart. He was very sincere and methodical in managing patients and keeping the record. Many stalwarts in the field of urology have contributed to this handbook and I am sure this will be of immense help to the postgraduates and practicing urologists. The material and the quality of the pictures and photographs are excellent.

**PN Dogra** MS MCh FAMS DSc (H)
Immediate Past President of Urological Society of India
Professor and Head, Department of Urology
All India Institute of Medical Sciences
New Delhi, India

# Preface

Transurethral endoscopic procedures have become as inherent part of urology. A thorough knowledge of the basics of transurethral endoscopy is necessary for a urologist. Though surgery is learnt in the operation theater, basic knowledge is essential for safe learning. This book will be helpful as a guide while endeavoring into uroendoscopy. Keeping in mind the need of the beginners of uroendoscopy, chapters have been designed to impart 'practical' knowledge of basic transurethral resection techniques to the readers. Chapters on endoscopic anatomy, instruments used for urethrocystoscopy, and patient preparation will be useful for beginners. The technique of resecting a prostatic chip is explained in detail. Transurethral resection of the prostate by unipolar and bipolar techniques has been described in separate chapters. Newer advancements like techniques of transurethral enucleation and resection, transurethral vaporization, holmium laser vaporization of the prostate have also been included. The surgical procedure is incomplete without postoperative care. Chapters on complications and postoperative care will give a comprehensive knowledge of uroendoscopy.

I convey my immense gratitude to the authors who have contributed to this book.

**M Anandan**

# Acknowledgments

I am grateful to the authors who have passed on their decades old wisdom to the readers by contributing the chapters.

I thank Arunkumar, Deepak Rathi, Ganesh Gopalakrishnan, R Manikandan, Mallikarjuna Chiruvella, RM Meyyappan, PVLN Murthy, Narmada P Gupta, K Senthil, N Selvarajan, and R Vijayakumar, for devoting their precious time and effort in drafting the chapters.

I thank M/s Jaypee Brothers Medical Publishers (P) Ltd, New Delhi, India, and their staff for providing all the necessary help in shaping of the book.

I convey my gratitude to my parents, wife and daughters for supporting me in bringing out this book.

I thank the Almighty for giving me the opportunity to edit this book.

# Contents

1. **Introduction and Brief History of Uroendoscopy**    1
   *M Anandan, C Ramesh*

2. **Endoscopes and Resection Instruments: Handling and Sterilization**    3
   *K Senthil*

3. **Diathermy and Lasers: A Resectionist Perspective**    12
   *M Anandan*

4. **Endoscopic Anatomy of the Urethra and Bladder**    18
   *M Anandan*

5. **Anesthesia for Transurethral Resection of Prostate and Transurethral Resection of Bladder Tumor**    27
   *N Selvarajan*

6. **Patient Preparation and Operation Theater Setup for Transurethral Resection**    34
   *M Anandan*

7. **Basics of Transurethral Resection**    39
   *M Anandan*

8. **Transurethral Monopolar Resection of the Prostate**    49
   *Ganesh Gopalakrishnan*

9. **Transurethral Enucleation and Resection of Prostate**    67
   *Mallikarjuna Chiruvella, Md Taif Bendigeri*

10. **Laser Enucleation and Vaporization of Prostate**    94
    *Arunkumar, R Vijayakumar*

11. **Transurethral Resection of Bladder Tumor**    102
    *RM Meyyappan*

12. **Bipolar Transurethral Resection of the Prostate**    115
    *Narmada P Gupta, Deepak Rathi*

13. **Postoperative Care Following Transurethral Resection of the Prostate** ........ 122
    *R Manikandan*

14. **Complications in Transurethral Resection of Prostate** ........ 127
    *PVLN Murthy*

*Index* ........ *139*

# Chapter 1

# Introduction and Brief History of Uroendoscopy

*M Anandan, C Ramesh*

## INTRODUCTION

The management of urological diseases has undergone a colossal change since the time Philipp Bozzini first visualized the interior of the bladder using a candle and lens. Now transurethral procedures and minimally invasive procedures, as such, have become sine qua non of urology practice. This necessitates the budding urologists to have a thorough basic knowledge of transurethral procedures at the beginning of their career.

The initial instrument designed by Bozzini—an obstetrician, used a wide mouthed funnel with its wide end attached to a lamp stand with beeswax candle. This "Lichtleiter" (1806) was cumbersome to use and not put into wide clinical practice. It was modified by Pierre Salomon Segalas (1826) to increase the illumination by using candles and mirror.

The "Father of cystoscopy", Antonin Jean Désormeaux (1953), a French urologist further modified it by replacing the candle with a lamp and first coined the word "endoscope". He performed the first transurethral procedure—removal of urethral papilloma. His instruments focused the brighter lamp light through multiple mirrors into the lumen with minimal loss of luminosity.

The next major breakthrough was the use of prisms and lenses in the endoscope by Nitze. This created a clearer and wider panoramic image. He also used a platinum loop light source at the tip of the scope for better illumination. The drawback of this design was the need for a cooling system for light source. This was further improved by the advent of tungsten incandescent lamp with better qualities and efficiencies.

Boisseau du Rocher modified the cystoscope to have components—the sheath and lens system. This helped in insertion of instruments like catheters through a channel. These "primitive" instruments were deemed functional by the development of resectoscope by Maximilian Stern in 1926. Prostate and bladder tumor resections became feasible.

Physicist Harold Hopkins brought in the next major advance in the endoscope era—the rod lens system of optics. He changed the optics by using long cylindrical rods with antireflection coatings as transmission medium and intervening small air columns as lenses. This produced clearer, brighter images. The discovery by Lamm that light can be transmitted through flexible glass fibers without loss of luminosity, helped in the development of fiber optics, flexible scopes and cold light sources.

Transurethral resections form majority of the uroendoscopic procedures. With benign prostatic hypertrophy being one of the most common urological problems affecting the elderly, transurethral resection of the prostate (TURP) forms the crux of urosurgical training. Review articles bring forth the fact that the average size of the gland subjected for TURP is increased, with the advent of alpha blockers and 5-alpha reductase inhibitors in the management of benign prostatic hyperplasia (BPH). Hence, better and safe resection practices are necessary for better patient outcome.

Newer modalities of "prostate ablation", other than electric current are available, like lasers, which have some benefits over the classical monopolar diathermy. They are useful in large prostates and in those with medical conditions that restrict the use of hypoosmolar irrigants during the procedure.

# Chapter 2

# Endoscopes and Resection Instruments: Handling and Sterilization

*K Senthil*

## INTRODUCTION

The progress in the field of urology as a specialty is in part due to the various instruments developed for endoscopic surgery. Knowledge of these instruments and their sterilization techniques is essential prior to starting endosurgery. Endoscopic surgery will be safe and comfortable only if performed using the appropriate and proper instruments and in the appropriate operation theater.

The operation theater should have sufficient moving space after the endoscopy cart along with the diathermy is positioned. Artificial lighting is preferable to sunlight. Sunlight can interfere with the vision of the monitor. Flooring and drainage of the irrigating fluid should be kept in mind while designing the operation theater. A funnel at the bottom end of the operating table will help the fluid to be channelled into a bucket or other drainage mechanism.

We should always remember that the diathermy can interfere with the ECG and hence should be placed in such a manner that there would be minimal or no interference.

Separate room for instrument laying; storage of instruments; cleansing and sterilization; and for anesthetic would be preferable.

## INSTRUMENTS

Transurethral resection involves a full set of special instruments as mentioned below.

*Cystoscope*—30° telescope is used for transurethral resection as only with a 30° telescope it is possible to view the prostatic lobes, bladder neck, resected tissue and the loop used for resection.

All the telescopes come with a Hopkins rod lens system. These have a wider angle of vision; brighter images as more light can be transmitted and the image resolution is better.

One has to note that the light pillar of each manufacturer varies and hence it is advisable to use the same system throughout. However adaptors for different light cables are available and hence telescopes of different manufacturers are interchangeable.

*Resectoscope sheath*—Several sizes of resectoscope sheaths are available. The sizes that are available commonly are 24 Fr, 26 Fr, 27 Fr and 28 Fr. 22 Fr resectoscope is also available and is used for narrow urethra. 22 Fr resectoscope sheath is coded white. 24 Fr and 26 Fr resectoscope sheath have the color code yellow and it fits the loops, which are yellow. Similarly, the resectoscopes sized 27 Fr and 28 Fr are coded black and they fit loops which are coded brown.

The oblique beak resectoscope is the most commonly used. Long beak and short beak resectoscopes are available but not used routinely as they have many disadvantages.

Resectoscopes sheath should be heat resistant, strong and a nonconductor of electricity. Hence they are now made of MTC which stands for metal, ceramic and teflon. Most of the sheath is metal. The beak has an inner coating of ceramic, which is nonconductor and heat resistant. The distal part is made of Teflon which is a nonconductor.

Resectoscope sheaths come with an inner sheath which helps in drainage of fluid—continuous irrigation Igelesias sheaths. This way the resection can be carried on for a longer period of time and the pressures in the bladder remains low during resection. Older resectoscopes used to be nonirrigation types which are not used commonly nowadays.

Some surgeons prefer to use the rotating resectoscopes which allow the surgeon to rotate the working element and telescope and resect all the lobes of the prostate without rotating the outer sheath in the urethra. These are less abrasive to the urethra and ergonomically more comfortable for the surgeon.

*Obturator*—Obturator is needed for introduction of the resectoscope sheath into the bladder. The safest way of introduction is the use of visual obturator where it is done entirely under vision (Schmidt obturator). Straight obturator and hinged obturator (timberlake) are introduced blindly with plenty of lubrication. The hinged obturator has a hinged angulation at the tip which can help to negotiate the bulbar urethra; bladder neck and if there is a large median lobe.

*Working element*—Working element is introduced and fixed to the resectoscope sheath once the resectoscope sheath is in the bladder.

The older version was the rack and pinion type which works by to and fro movement. This type of working element is difficult master.

The commonly used type of working element are the thumb operated (Nesbit system) and the finger operated (Baumrucker system).

In the thumb-operated system, the loop stays within the sheath in the resting state. The loop is extended out of the sheath by pressure and the spring helps to pull it back. As the cutting happens without any pressure and by the action of the spring this system is named as passive. This can be used for optical internal urethrotomy as well. The cutting can be slower than the active loop.

In the finger-operated system, the loop is outside the resectoscope sheath at rest and it is important not to activate the current accidentally. Cutting is done by actively drawing the loop into the sheath.

*Loops for resection*—Appropriate loops are used as per the size of the resectoscope sheath. The loops are also color-coded as per the resectoscope sheath.

Standard loop is 0.35 mm. Thin loop is 0.25 mm thick and thick loop is 0.40 mm thick. Thin loop needs less current and hence causes less charring. They are used for precise cutting without char like in a bladder tumor. Thick loop is used for resecting the prostatic lobes. Over a period of time after several uses the thick loops become thin.

Several types of loops are available. Standard cutting loop is the most versatile loop, which can be singly used for many purposes like cutting and coagulation. Roller ball electrode is used for coagulation after resection. Collins knife is used to do a bladder neck incision. These are the commonly used loops. Others like conical electrode are used for point coagulation. Blunt and sharp curettes are used for scraping adherent slough or necrotic tissue.

*Diathermy cable*—Two types of high frequency cables are available. Single stem cable fits on top of the working element and double stem cable fits at the bottom of the working element. The double stem electrode can be exposed to the irrigation fluid more easily and hence can get short circuited occasionally.

*Diathermy equipment*—Good diathermy is a vital equipment for resection to be carried out. A stand by diathermy will be a valuable asset if available.

*Light source and cable*—Halogen, xenon and LED light sources are available. LED light sources are being used more widely than before nowadays. They provide a "whiter" light, similar to sunlight so that the colors are clearly deciphered.

*Irrigation tubes*—Disposable irrigation tubes are readily available. Suitable tube providing adequate flow should be selected.

*Evacuator*—Once the resection is complete, evacuator is used to wash out the prostatic chips in the bladder. Elliks evacuator has two glass bulbs connected to a rubber bulb and connector. Disposable modified plastic Elliks evacuator is also available.

Some surgeons use Toomey syringe for evacuation. Toomey syringe is a glass syringe with a metal tip adapter to fix to the resectoscope sheath. It is very useful for evacuation of clots. Active suctioning effect is used in Toomy syringe and passive suctioning effect is used in Ellick's evacuator.

*Sieve*—A sieve is used to filter out the prostatic chips from the evacuator. The collected chips are sent for histopathological examination.

*Drainage hose*—Some centers use a drainage hose to drain the outflowing irrigation fluid.

*Instruments to be available as standby*:
- Meatotomy scissors
- Otis urethrotome
- Internal urethrotomy and vesicolithotripsy equipment
- Biopsy forceps

*Bipolar resection*—Bipolar resection involves plasma arc for cutting the tissue. It uses a different working element, loop and diathermy equipment which is not the same as for the monopolar resection. The advantage of bipolar technology is that the irrigating fluid is saline and there is no risk of TUR syndrome.

## STERILIZATION

Success and safety of the surgery depends a lot on sterilization. Unlike open surgical instruments, endoscopic instruments are more intricate and delicate and hence need special care during cleaning and sterilization.

All major centers have a standardized process for sterilization and monitoring of the process of sterilization. Only the trained personnel should be authorized to handle the instruments and carry out the sterilization process.

The instruments should never be stacked or kept one on top of the other at any stage of cleansing or sterilization. Delicate optics and instruments can be permanently damaged by dropping them accidentally. The light cable and cable of cameras should be loosely coiled to prevent damage.

The process of sterilization starts with cleansing. Endoscopic instruments should not be left to dry after the procedure. If it is not possible to clean the instruments soon after the procedure they may be soaked in water till that time. The instruments are dismantled completely before they are soaked.

Blood clots, charring and tissue debris can be stuck to the surface and to the irrigation channels and sieves. Organic material may be cleansed using neutral pH enzymatic detergents. The enzymatic cleansers may be temperature sensitive and hence instructions should be adhered to. Mechanical cleansing or ultrasonic cleansing is not suitable for endoscopic instruments as they may cause scratches and dents and remove lubricants. Abrasives which are used for open instruments should be avoided. Lenses are cleaned with 70% alcohol-based solutions.

The cystoscope and resectoscope sheaths are autoclavable and can be steam sterilized. If there are time constraints, chemical sterilization using gluteraldehyde is used.

Cystoscope is one of the most delicate instrument and should be handled with at most care. The surface of the telescope should be inspected for evidence of burns, scratches and dents. Vision should be checked after every procedure and if found to be hazy, the first step would be to clean the tip with cleansing agent and neutral pH enzymatic cleaning solution detergent.

Inner sheath and outer sheath should be disassembled and separately cleaned. The stopcocks should be opened and cleaned and if necessary disassembled to make sure that there is no debris or clot.

Once the instruments are cleaned they are sterilized as per the policy in the institution. Steam sterilization of endoscopes is not advisable unless it is specified as autoclavable in the user manual. It varies depending on the manufacturer. It is always better to adhere to the technique advised by the manufacturer for adequate and safe sterilization.

Glutaraldehyde is a virucidal, fungicidal, bactericidal and sporicidal agent used at 2.4% or 3.5% concentrations. 2.4% solution without surfactant is suitable for endoscopic instruments. Glutaraldehyde is a caustic agent and hence has to be thoroughly washed off the instruments prior to use. The personnel handling it also should take proper precautions. Contact period recommended for undiluted 2.4% glutaraldehyde solution is 45 minutes at 25°C (77°F). For 0.55% ortho-phthalaldehyde (e.g. CIDEX OPA) contact period is 12 minutes at 20°C (68°F) or higher. STERRAD® is a plasma or vapor phase sterilizer, and can also be used for endoscope sterilization.

Gas sterilization using ethylene oxide is an effective method of sterilization followed in many centers. The sterilization takes about one-and-half hour. It is important to aerate the sterilized equipment at least for 8–12 hours so that the gas gets eluded.

Light cable and camera cannot be sterilized and hence would need a sterile disposable cover.

It is very important to remember that we should not reuse accessories termed as single use only.

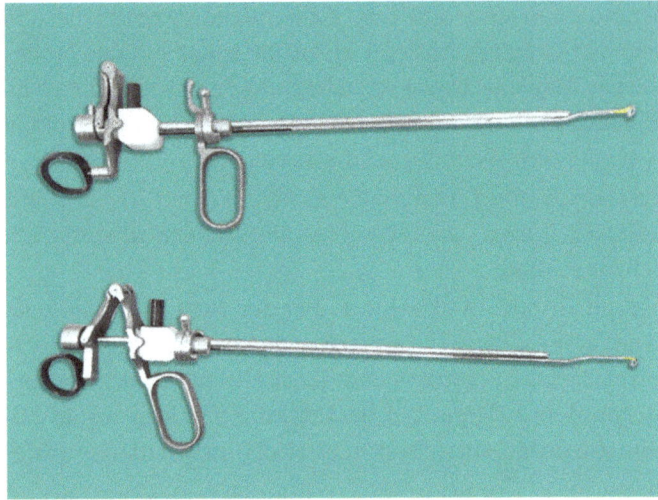

Thumb operated (Above) and Finger operated (Below) working elements.

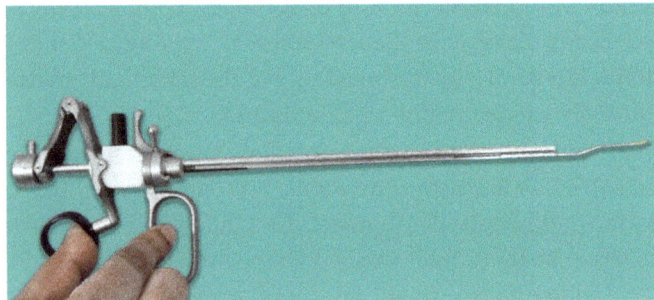

Thumb-operated working element.

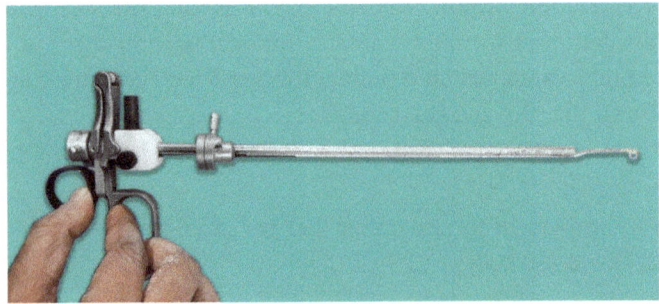

Finger-operated working element.

# Endoscopes and Resection Instruments: Handling and Sterilization

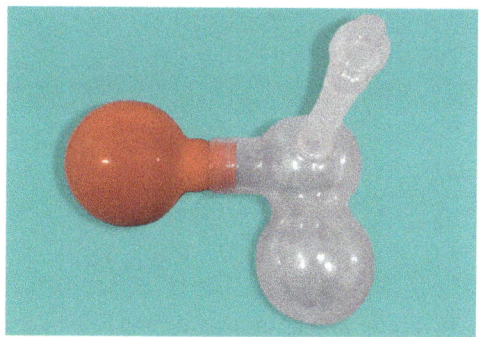

Ellick's evacuator.

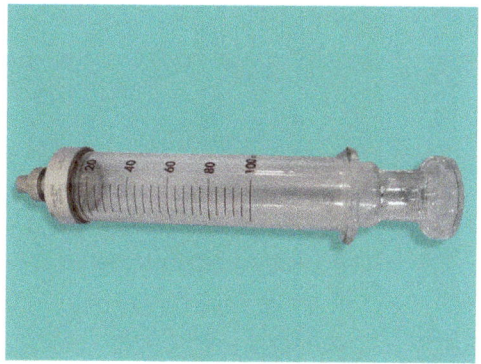

Toomeys' syringe.

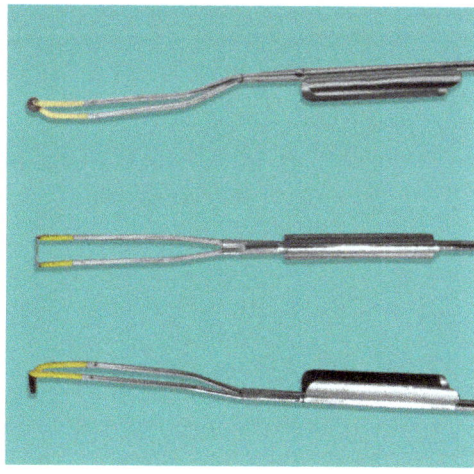

Electrodes:
1. Rollerball electrode
2. Loop electrode
3. Collin's incision knife.

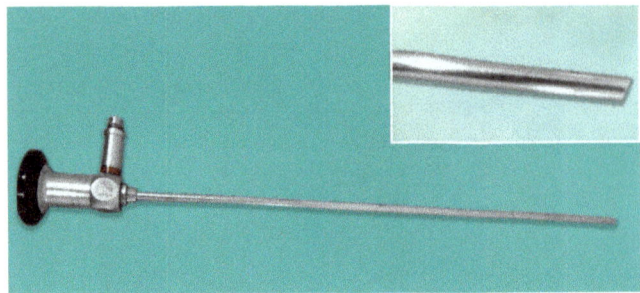

30° Scope with inset showing angulated tip.

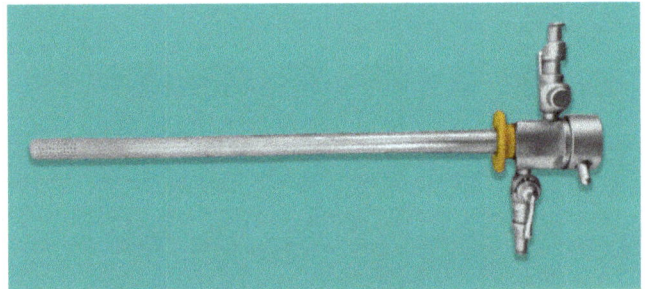

Outer sheath of resectoscope.

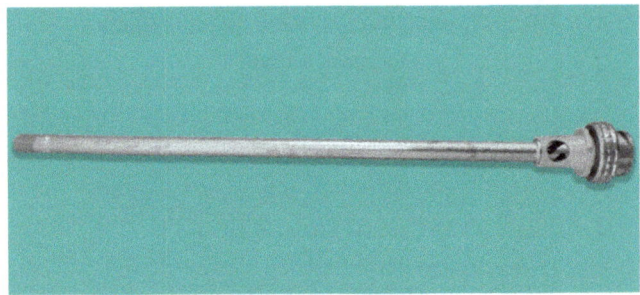

Inner sheath of resectoscope.

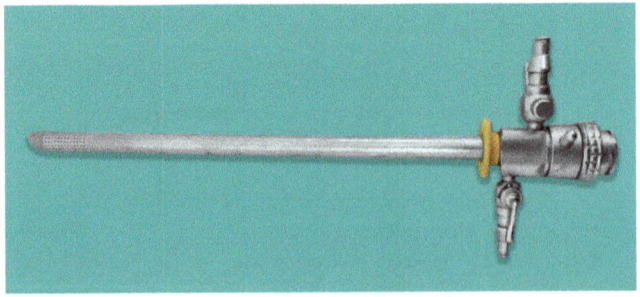

Completed sheath assembly of resectoscope.

# Endoscopes and Resection Instruments: Handling and Sterilization 11

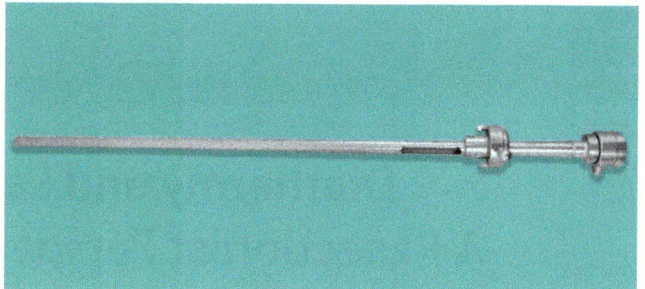

Visual obturator.

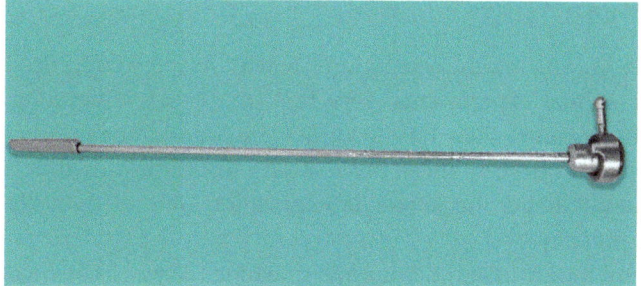

Blind obturator.

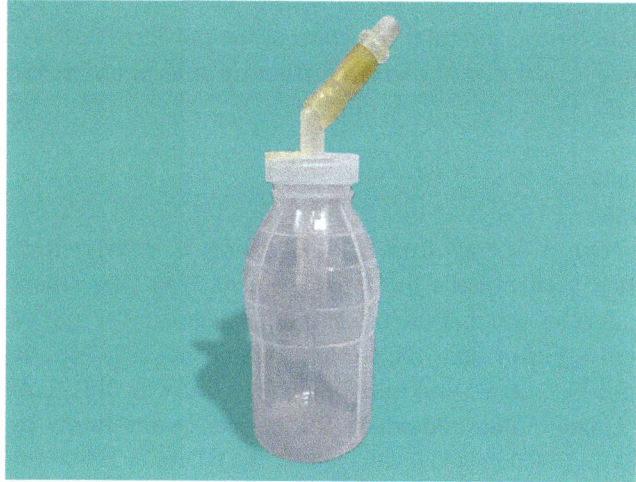

Ellick's evacuator.

# Chapter 3

# Diathermy and Lasers: A Resectionist Perspective

*M Anandan*

## INTRODUCTION

Diathermy is one of the inventions which has revolutionized surgery. Based on animal experiments, very high frequency alternating currents, with frequency more than 100–200 kHz were found to be nonexcitatory for the muscles and nerves. These did not alter the cardiac rhythm either. The reason for this being the longer repolarization time of the cells than the current frequency.

The commonly used diathermy machines have frequencies in the range of 0.2–3.3 MHz. This gives a good safety margin to avoid accidental stimulations. The diathermy machines also differ on their power, varying from 50 watts to 400 watts. Typically, surgeries requiring under water cutting need higher power. Machines with 300 watts to 400 watts power are preferred for transurethral resection of the prostate (TURP).

The three mechanisms by which diathermy units or electrosurgery units function are:
1. Cutting
2. Coagulation
3. Fulguration.

The electrical energy from the electrode is converted to thermal energy when it encounters the impedance of body. The amount of heat generated decides whether the tissue is cut, coagulated or fulgurated. If the temperature is higher than 100°C, water within the cells vaporize and the cell ruptures like a blast and membrane breaks down. This "cuts" into the tissues to create the desired effect. The frequency waveforms are typically continuous and relatively low voltage (Fig. 3.1). During TURP, cutting is the main mode used to resect the prostate chips. The current concentration is inversely proportional to the thickness of the loop. Hence, thinner loops are better for cutting.

If the temperature is between 65°C and 90°C, the proteins become denatured and form a coagulum. If the coagulum forms within the blood

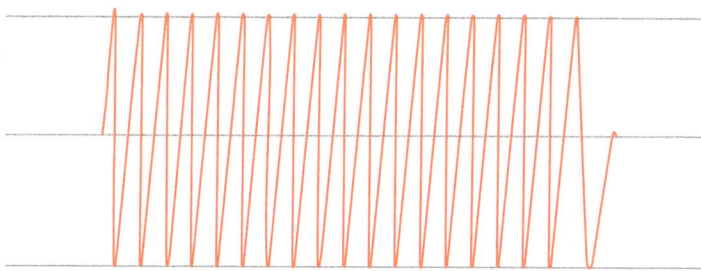

**Fig. 3.1:** Continuous waveforms of cutting current.

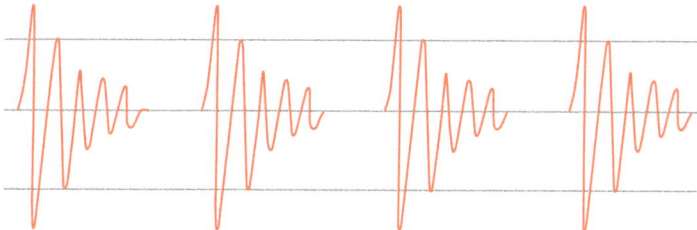

**Fig. 3.2:** Intermittent pulse waveforms of coagulation mode current.

vessels, the bleeding stops. The other method to stop bleeding is to compress the blood vessels and allow approximation of both the walls of the vessel with a sticky coagulum. This coagulation effect is rendered by the application of current in bursts with high voltage, rather than the continuous form with the cutting current. Coagulation mode is used for control of large arterial and venous bleeders during resection. Thicker loops (the sides of the loop) are better for coagulation (Fig. 3.2).

The third type is the fulguration, where the tissue is not in contact with the electrode. Here electric sparks are generated with very high temperatures of more than 400°C. In such situations, the layer of tissue is "burnt" due to the carbonization of the proteins, sugars and nucleic acids resulting in the formation of carbonized black layer at the surface. Fulguration is useful for diffuse oozing from the prostate surface. Ball electrode uses the fulguration and coagulation principle combined, for better hemostasis.

Any electrical circuit should be completed, for functioning. From the generator, the current circuit should return to the ground or the neural plate. Depending on the whether the current returns through the body or through the second lead, it is categorized as monopolar or bipolar respectively. Since the second lead is closeby, the current dissipation is minimal with bipolar diathermy. This is explained in the picture. Monopolar diathermy requires the neutral plate, which is not absolutely necessary with bipolar instruments (Figs. 3.3 and 3.4). The bipolar diathermy is relatively safer for those with pacemaker since there is transmission of current through the body. The stimulation of nerves and is also minimal with bipolar diathermy.

The plasmakinetic resection is a special kind of bipolar resection. In this form of resection, a cloud of plasma is formed around the bipolar loop on activation. This heats up the tissues, vaporizes and cuts them. The main

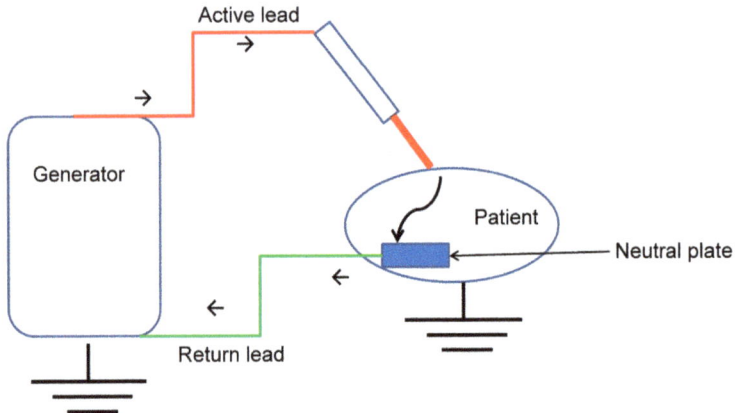

**Fig. 3.3:** Monopolar circuit—circuit completed through the patient body and the neutral plate.

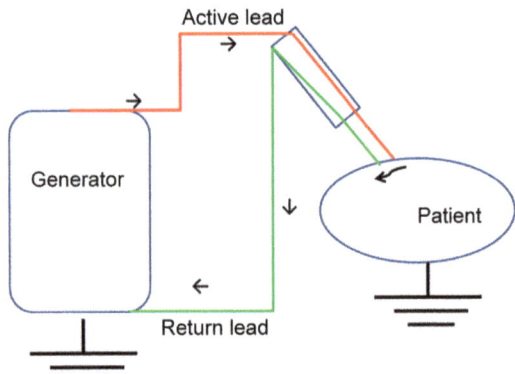

**Fig. 3.4:** Bipolar circuit. Note that the patient is not forming the transmission part in the circuit.

effect is local concentrated locally. There is no gross dispersion of current and minimal collateral damage.

The most important patient safety drill in diathermy is the foolproof fixation of neutral plate. The neutral plate provides a wide area of current transfer, so that the heat generated is minimal. The few points to be noted are:
- It should close to the area of surgery—preferably in the thigh, mid-calf, or below buttocks for transurethral surgeries
- The area should be scarless, hairless
- Should not be fixed over bony prominences
- Full contact with skin necessary, partial contact can cause burns
- There should not be any metal contact with the patient's body before between the neutral plate and surgical field.

## LASERS

LASER is the abbreviation of "light amplification by stimulated emission of radiation". Laser devices convert electrical energy into light energy. The laser device has three components—(1) the excitation source, (2) the medium and (3) the resonator system. The excitation source produces electrical flash which induces the electrons in the medium into activated state and release photon. This is concentrated into a coherent beam by the resonator. This produces monochromatic, coherent collimated laser beam. Depending upon the medium used, which could be solid, liquid or gas, different wavelengths of lasers are produced, with different effects.

The effect of laser on tissues depends on the reflection, scattering, or absorption of the beam. Reflection causes unintended damage to surrounding tissues and scattering diffuses the beam. The main effect is caused by absorption, which converts light energy to thermal energy. This results in either coagulation or vaporization depends on the temperature reached, similar to diathermy. The main laser energy absorbants of relevance in the prostate tissue are water and oxyhemoglobin. Depending on the variability of laser absorption by these two components, the different lasers have different effects. The more transparent tissues (with less vascularity and hemoglobin) lead to deeper penetration of laser and vice versa. This is depicted as absorption coefficient of tissue. The higher the absorption coefficient, more opaque the tissues are.

The depth of penetration also depends on the wavelength of the lasers. Beams with shorter wavelengths travel shorter distances. The laser intensity, and not the duration of application determine the vaporization. Similar to diathermy, coagulated tissues prevent further penetration of the laser beams.

Similar to the current waves in diathermy, lasers can be continuous or pulsed lasers. Pulsed wave has more precision and less lateral heat conduction. This minimizes damage to surrounding tissues. The commonly used lasers are Nd:YAG, Ho:YAG, KTP:YAG, Tm:YAG and diode lasers for prostate.

*Nd:YAG laser*: These lasers have a wavelength of 1,064 nm. It has low absorption coefficient and hence has a tissue penetration of more than 1 cm. Both water and hemoglobin do not absorb these lasers effectively. This causes more coagulative necrosis and is more effective in coagulating the tissues rather than vaporizing or cutting them. Though it was the initial laser used for prostate, it is uncommonly used now due to its inefficiencies. After the prostate surface is coagulated, a necrotic area is formed, which may take days to weeks for sloughing off. Till then patient may experience severe voiding and storage symptoms.

*Ho:YAG laser*: This is commonly used for prostatectomy. It is a pulsed solid-state laser with a 2,140 nm wavelength and pulse duration of 350 ms. It is well absorbed by water (and tissues with water) and hence heat is dispersed fast. Depth of penetration is 0.4 mm. It causes vaporization of tissues since prostate has high water content and large amount of energy is absorbed. The thermal damage is limited to 0.5–1.0 mm. It is a contact type laser requiring contact of the tip of the fiber with the tissue for activation. Minimal dissipating heat of 2–3 mm helps vessel coagulation.

*KTP:YAG laser*: This is produced by passing Nd:YAG laser beam through KTP crystal. The wavelength is 532 nm giving a greenish yellow light. It is selectively absorbed by hemoglobin and *not* by water. The penetration depth is 0.8 mm and the system is quasi continuous wave laser with pulses less than 0.25 s. Since the laser is absorbed by hemoglobin, lesser beam penetrates the tissues and blood filled prostate tissue is vaporized rapidly with a 1.0 mm rim of coagulation. Since it is more active in hemoglobin, it is better suited for hemostasis.

*Tm:YAG laser*: It is a continuous wave with wavelength of 2,000 nm. It is well absorbed by water. The depth of penetration is 0.25 nm. Its use is similar to that of Holmium lasers.

*Diode lasers* use a special diode for energy generation. Various wavelengths are available—940 nm, 980 nm or 1,470 nm. These are absorbed by both water and hemoglobin and hence have good vaporization and coagulation. Since less thermal waste is induced during diode laser induction, the cooling systems are comparatively smaller than the other lasers and hence the machine is compact.

The laser fibers are designed with different delivery methods. It could be (1) end firing with bare tip or sculptured tip, (2) side firing with metal or glass reflector and prismatic internal reflector, (3) interstitial with bare tip, diffuser tip or diffuser tip with temperature transducer.

Side firing is used in Nd:YAG and KTP lasers which are applied to the surface of the prostate, usually without direct contact, resulting in necrosis of the prostate layer by layer. KTP laser causes vaporization and Nd:YAG laser causes coagulation. Holmium lasers are contact lasers which are effective on direct contact with the prostate since they have less depth of penetration. Nd:YAG and KTP lasers have been tried as interstitial lasers, with the fiber inserted into the prostate and forming an area of coagulation necrosis around the tip.

Lasers are generally preferred for the patients on antiplatelets and anticoagulants, and also those with cardiac risks, who may not tolerate fluid overload caused by irrigant fluids.

# Chapter 4

# Endoscopic Anatomy of the Urethra and Bladder

*M Anandan*

## INTRODUCTION

The operating surgeon should have a thorough knowledge of the surgical anatomy for successful surgical practice. This holds good for open surgery, endoscopic surgery and laparoscopic/robotic surgery. The anatomical knowledge of the structures and organs we encounter during our procedure helps in decreasing the complications and also helps in the successful completion of the procedure.

The surgeon starting the transurethral resection procedures need to know the important landmarks he would encounter during the procedures and also the nearby structures which could get injured during the procedure. The common variations from the normal anatomy should also be known. Intraoperative mishaps during endoscopic procedures are comparatively more difficult to manage than during open procedures, since the vision is affected due to the bleeding or otherwise.

The "resectionist" needs to know the anatomy of the urethra, prostate, and the bladder mucosa with its variations.

## ANATOMY OF THE URETHRA

The urethra starts form the external urethral meatus and ends at the bladder neck. The "prostate" visualized by endoscope is actually the prostatic urethra with the bulge caused by prostate gland invading the urethral "space".

### Meatus

The external urethral meatus is a longitudinal slit located in the glans slightly ventral to the midline. The normal urethral meatus is 24–26 Fr. size. Urethral meatus may be calibrated using urethral dilators to 26 Fr so that the standard resectoscope can be inserted without force.

Navicular fossa is the dilated part of the urethra just proximal to the meatus. This part is usually poorly documented during rigid cystoscopy since the flow of the irrigant through the bevelled ends prevents adequate distension of the urethra at this part.

## Penile Urethra

The penile urethra is the next anatomical structure seen by endoscopy. This part of the urethra is characterized by plexiform, irregularly oriented blood vessels. The urethra is *without* any curvature, forming a straight tunnel if the penis is held stretched. Multiple small punctate elevated spots can be seen in longitudinal orientation. These correspond to the opening of the Litter's glands (Figs. 4.1 and 4.2). The mucosa is pink. There may be areas of white thickenings or narrowing signifying strictures. In some occasions, if local anesthetic jelly is instilled with force, small petechial hemorrhagic spots may be seen.

## Bulbar Urethra

Bulbar urethra starts from the penoscrotal junction. Endoscopically it can be identified by the change in the orientation of the blood vessels—from the plexiform to longitudinal orientation. The urethra is comparatively roomier and a gentle curvature is seen rather than the straight penile urethra (Fig. 4.3).

## Membranous Urethra (External Urethral Sphincter)

The bulbar urethra ends in the membranous urethra (external urethral sphincter, Fig. 4.4). This is seen at the termination of the curvature of the bulbar urethra (endoscope oriented down to up, with the scope between

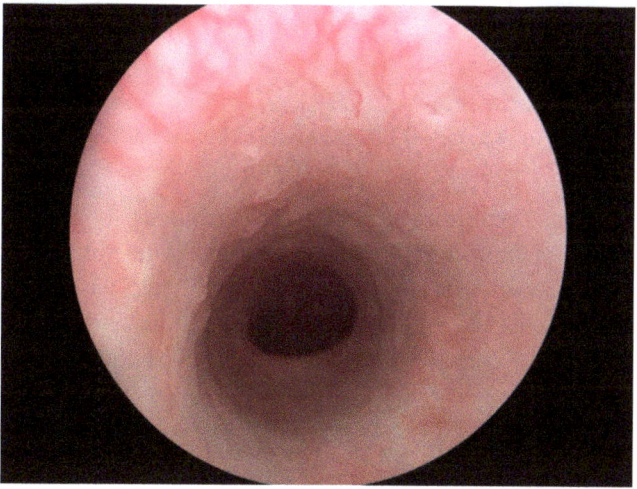

**Fig. 4.1:** Litter's glands.

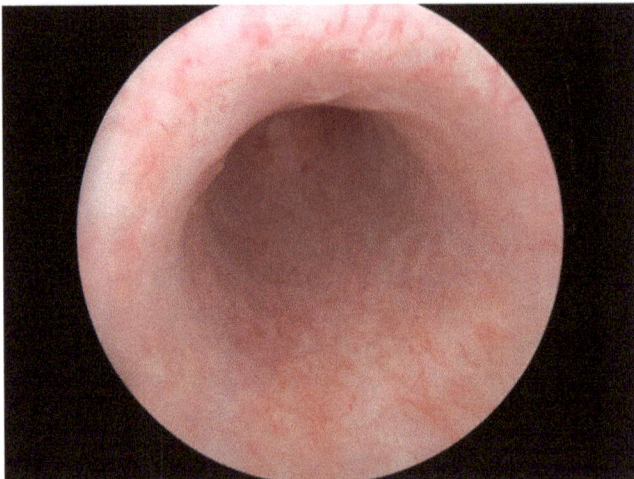

**Fig. 4.2:** Plexiform blood vessels of penile urethra.

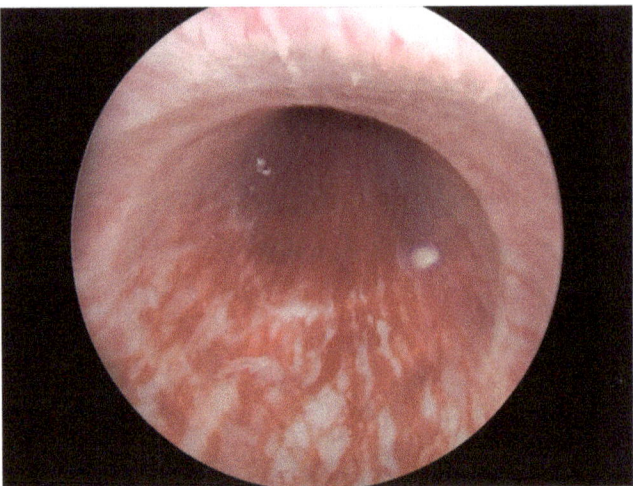

**Fig. 4.3:** Linear blood vessels of bulbar urethra.

the thighs when seen from outside). The sphincter is seen as radially oriented ridges in centrifugal appearance. Usually the sphincter is closed, especially if done under local anesthesia. A small "tug" with the scope over the sphincter will usually elicit sphincter contraction. Wide open sphincter indicates atonic sphincter or complete muscle relaxation.

## Verumontanum

Proximal to the sphincter, verumontanum is seen as a small projection located dorsally in the prostatic urethra. The prostatic utricle opens at the top

# Endoscopic Anatomy of the Urethra and Bladder

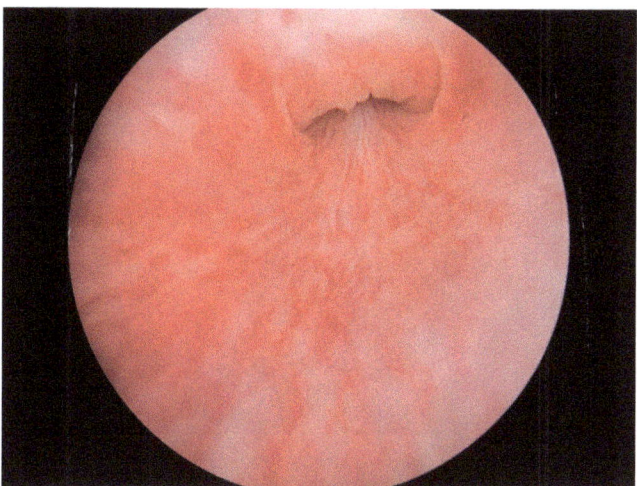

**Fig. 4.4:** External urethral sphincter.

of the verumontanum. The size of the opening is variable. Verumontanum is an important landmark, since the sphincter is located distal to it. Anatomically, the verumontanum is located in the center of the prostatic urethra. But, due to the differential enlargement of the prostate, the veru is pushed toward the apex of the prostate. Rarely veru can be flattened and its identification might be difficult.

## Prostatic Urethra

Normal prostatic urethra is roomy with 28-30 Fr caliber. Inward bulging of the prostate corresponds to enlarged prostate. Various grading systems are available to document the enlargement of the prostate. The simple grading for the lateral lobes usually practiced is as follows:
- Grade 1—Inward bulging of the prostate with both lobes away even without irrigation (Fig. 4.5)
- Grade 2—Both lobes touching each other without irrigation, but move away with irrigant flow (Figs. 4.6A and B)
- Grade 3—Both lobes touching each other even with irrigation (Fig. 4.7).

The grading for median lobe is:
- Grade 1—Trigone easily seen from the bladder neck with minimal tilt the scope
- Grade 2—Trigone seen with difficulty with huge angulation of scope
- Grade 3—Trigone cannot be seen.

The grading of the prostatic enlargement helps to assess the possible duration of resection, estimating blood loss and the need for suprapubic trocar. For grade 3 enlargement, other options like open prostatectomy, staged TURP, Holep should be considered.

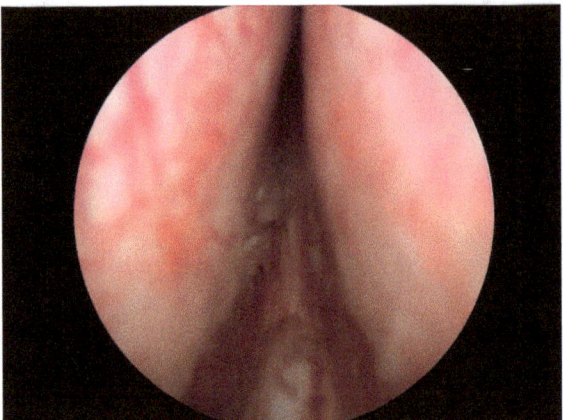

**Fig. 4.5:** Grade 1 lateral lobes of prostate.

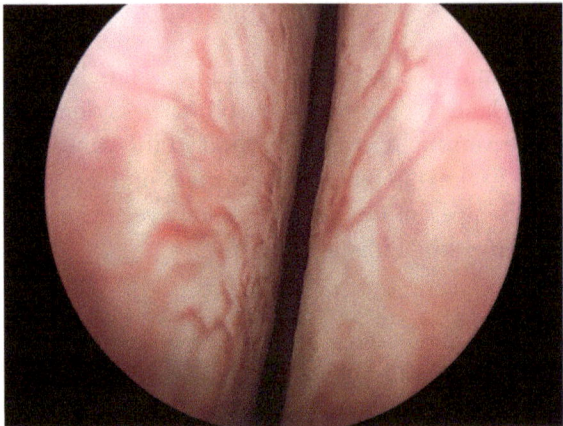

**Fig. 4.6A:** Grade 2 lateral lobes with flow on.

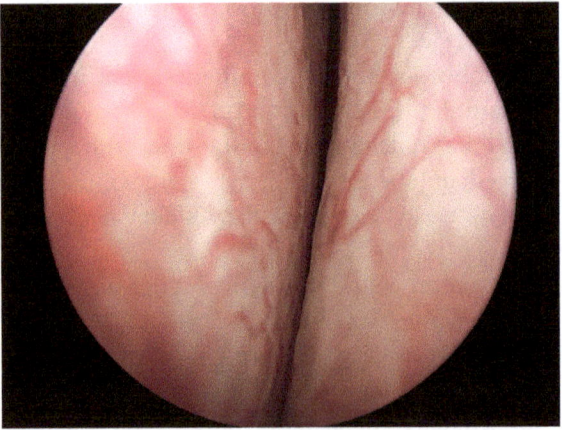

**Fig. 4.6B:** Grade 2 lateral lobes, with flow off.

# Endoscopic Anatomy of the Urethra and Bladder

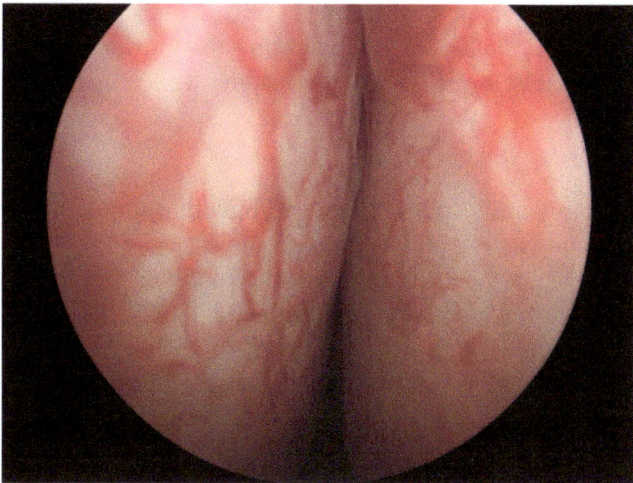

**Fig. 4.7:** Grade 3 lateral lobes with flow on.

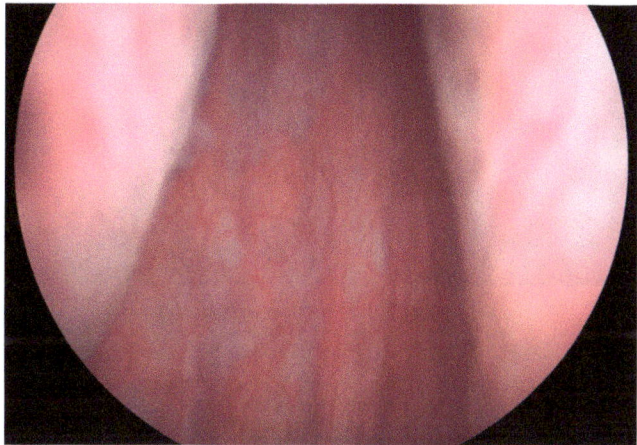

**Fig. 4.8:** Severe bladder neck elevation—Bladder neck aperture not seen from veru—Note the normal prostate gland lateral lobes.

## BLADDER NECK

Bladder neck comprises of the annular oriented detrusor fibers at the bladder outlet. In normal individuals, with the scope tip at the level of veru, bladder interior should be seen. The trigone and ureteric orifices should be visible with none or minimal tilt of the scope from the bladder neck.

We consider minimal bladder neck elevation, if bladder interior is partially seen from the veru, and severe elevation, if it is not seen at all (Fig. 4.8).

The differentiation of bladder neck and median lobe is that, in the former, there is a "shelf" or "wall" forming the barrier, whereas median lobe forms a mound at the level of the bladder neck (Fig. 4.9).

## BLADDER MUCOSA

Bladder mucosa is uniformly smooth and pink in normal individuals. Few prominent blood vessels are usual observations (Fig. 4.10).

Trabeculations are caused by the hypertrophy of the detrusor muscle bundles. They do not have any conformal orientation. They are associated

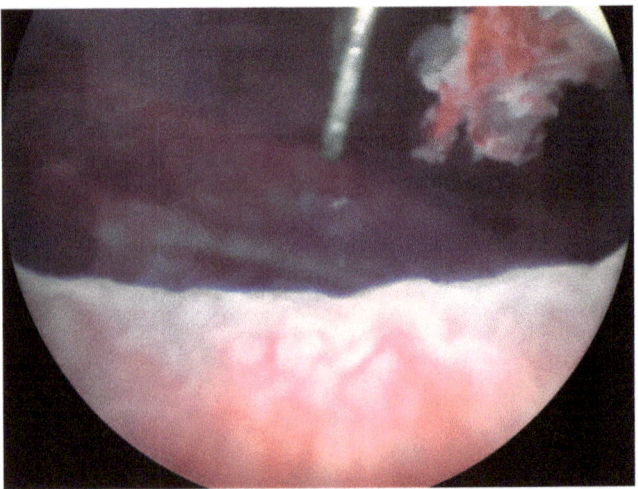

**Fig. 4.9:** Shelf like elevation of bladder neck.

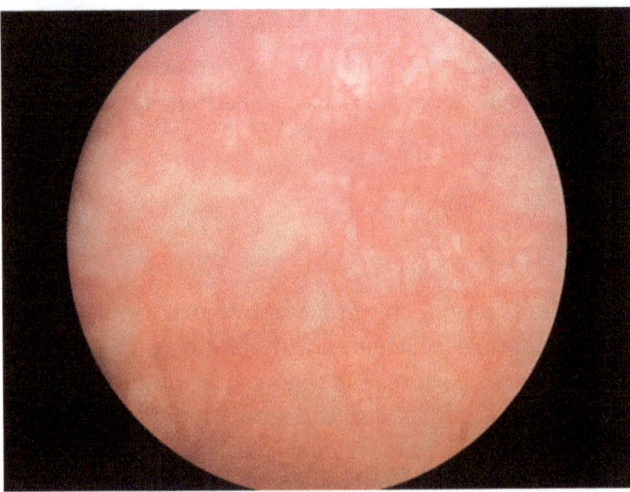

**Fig. 4.10:** Normal bladder mucosa.

# Endoscopic Anatomy of the Urethra and Bladder

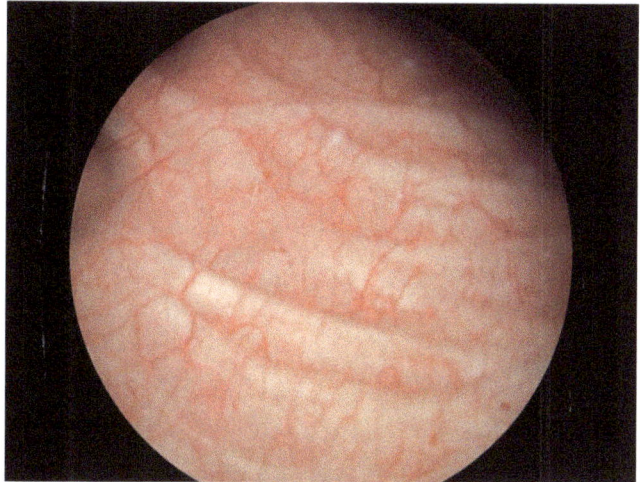

**Fig. 4.11:** Grade 1 trabeculations.

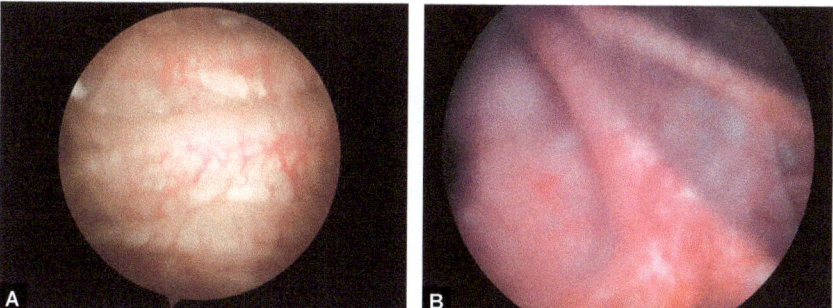

**Figs. 4.12A and B:** Grade 2 trabeculations.

with either anatomic or functional obstruction of bladder outlet. The trabeculations are classified into three grades:
1. Grade 1: Predominantly cellules (Fig. 4.11)
2. Grade 2: Predominantly saccules (Figs. 4.12A and B)
3. Grade 3: Presence of diverticulae (Figs. 4.13A and B)

Cellules, saccules and diverticulae are the mucosal outpouchings in between the trabeculations:
- *Cellules*: Outpouchings where the mucosa completely illuminates
- *Saccules*: Presence shadowing of the mucosa close to the muscle bundles
- *Diverticulae*: Mucosal outpouchings almost completely unilluminated, except when the scope is placed close to them.

In patients on indwelling catheters, mucosal bullous edema is seen mainly in the posterior and posterosuperior wall. This is due to the foreign body reaction caused by the catheter.

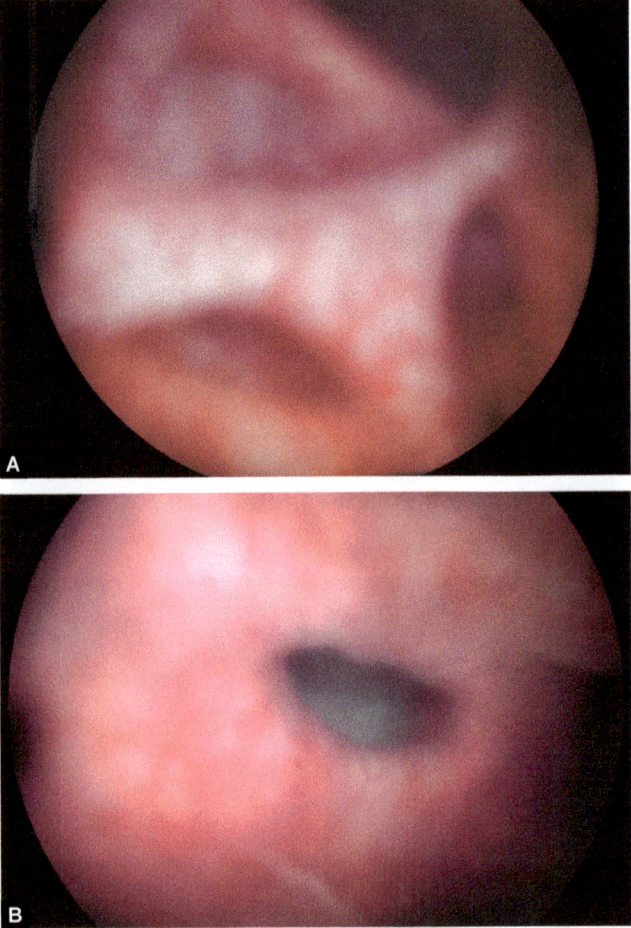

**Figs. 4.13A and B:** Grade 3 trabeculations.

## URETERIC ORIFICES

Ureteric orifices are difficult to identify in those with grade 2/3 trabeculations and those with grade 3 median lobes. The technique is to trace the Mercier's bar either from one of the ureteric orifices or from the midline and trace it along the bar.

# Chapter 5

# Anesthesia for Transurethral Resection of Prostate and Transurethral Resection of Bladder Tumor

*N Selvarajan*

## INTRODUCTION

Benign prostatic hyperplasia is common in males of over 60 years of age. This age group is associated with a lot of preexisting diseases like hypertension, diabetes mellitus, ischemic heart disease, respiratory diseases [chronic obstructive pulmonary disease (COPD), bronchial asthma and bronchitis] and renal impairment [secondary to hypertension (HT), diabetes mellitus (DM) or obstructive uropathy]. In some instances, these diseases are identified only during preanesthetic assessment. Though regional anesthesia (spinal or epidural anesthesia) is generally considered safer than general anesthesia, decision on the type of anesthesia has to be based on individualized risk assessment.

The regional anesthesia acts by blocking the sensory innervations of the prostate. The spinal segments involved in the neural innervation of the prostate and bladder neck is as follows:
- Sympathetic                              T11-L2,3
- Parasympathetic                          S2-4
- Spinal levels of pain conduction         T11-L2 and S2-4

Due to the ramification of the nerves in the pelvic plexus all these levels need to be blocked for adequate pain control. Prostate capsule is closely appended with thin-walled venous sinuses, which are directly communicating with the internal iliac veins.

## PREOPERATIVE ASSESSMENT

### History

Patient should be enquired about past anesthesia, surgery, comorbid conditions, allergies, treatment and drugs he is on.

### Drug Intake

Some drugs need special care and they may need to be stopped or continued during the perioperative period.

*Beta Blockers*: Beta blockers should not be stopped and should be continued till the time of surgery as they give protection against perioperative myocardial infarction. The compensatory tachycardiac response to fall in BP from spinal anesthesia and hemorrhage is obtunded by beta blockers.

*ACE inhibitors and angiotensin II receptor blockers*: Renin-angiotensin mediated response to hypovolemia may be impaired causing severe hypotension which may not respond to IV fluids. Hence these agents should be withheld on the day of surgery.

Alpha blockers also will cause hypotension but can be managed with IV fluids.

*Anticoagulants*: Apart from increasing the surgical bleeding, anticoagulants may cause serious spinal hematoma after spinal epidural or anesthesia. The INR should be less than 1.5 before going ahead with surgery. In emergency cases, adequate fresh frozen plasma (FFP) should be given to normalize the coagulation before surgery.

*Insulin and oral hypoglycemic agent (OHAs)*: These should not be given on the day of surgery for the fear of hypoglycemia. To control blood sugar plain insulin may be given IV in the perioperative period. Fasting blood sugar and serum potassium should be done on the day of surgery in patients on insulin. If required plain insulin may be given on the day of surgery. Patients on insulin, fasting blood sugar and potassium are to be done on the day of surgery.

## Cardiovascular System (CVS) Assessment

Recent onset poorly controlled heart failure is associated with high perioperative mortality. HT, DM, smoking, dyslipidemia and family history are the main risk factors for perioperative cardiac events.

The common anticoagulants and antiplatelets are used and the guidelines for duration of discontinuation are detailed in Table 5.1.

**Table 5.1:** Details of common anticoagulants and antiplatelets as well as the guidelines for duration of discontinuation.

| Drug group | Drug | Discontinue before | Antidote |
|---|---|---|---|
| NSAIDs | Aspirin | No need to stop before surgery | Platelets |
| Thienopyridines | • Clopidogrel<br>• Ticlopidine | 5–7 days<br>14 days | Platelets |
| GIIb/IIIa antagonists | | 4 weeks | Platelets |
| Low molecular weight heparins | Single dose<br>Twice daily dose | 12 hours<br>24 hours | FFP |
| Anticoagulants | Warfarin, acitrom | 3 days (PT/INR < 1.5) | FFP, Vitamin K |
| Unfractionated heparin IV | | 4 hours | Protamine/FFP |

(NSAIDs, nonsteroidal anti-inflammatory drugs; FFP: fresh frozen plasma)

- Aspirin 75 mg may be continued till surgery without much issues. But 150 mg aspirin dose must be stopped prior to surgery.
- Anticoagulants like warfarin should be stopped at least 3 days before and PT/INR checked. INR should not be more than 1.5 before taking up for surgery.

### Respiratory System

Patients who have severe cough, COPD or bronchial asthma may not be good candidates for spinal anesthesia. These patients may need further assessment by a pulmonologist to optimize the patient.

## INVESTIGATIONS

- Hemogram
- Random blood sugar
- Serum creatinine
- Serum electrolytes
- ECG for patients over 40 years and symptomatic patients
- Grouping and crossmatching when blood loss is anticipated
- Prothrombin time (PT/INR) if on anticoagulants
- Urinalysis
- Urine culture and sensitivity
- Pulmonary function test (PFT)—occasionally
- Arterial blood gas analysis (ABG)—rarely

## FASTING GUIDELINES

Starvation ensures an empty stomach and minimizes the chances for vomiting, regurgitation and aspiration. Strict adherence is necessary irrespective of the type of anesthesia, because "failed spinal" may end up in general anesthesia.

Six hours of starvation is necessary for solid foods, liquids containing milk, or fruit juices with pulp. Patient may take water or clear liquids about 2–3 hours before surgery. (Clear liquids—one should be able to read newspaper print through the glass containing that liquid).

## ANESTHETIC MANAGEMENT

### Spinal Anesthesia

Spinal anesthesia is the anesthesia of choice. The discomfort caused by bladder distension requires a sensory level up to T10 and this level provides

adequate relaxation for the surgeon. The advantages of spinal over general anesthesia are:
- Under spinal the blood loss is less necessitating fewer transfusions.
- The stress response is also reduced.
- As the patients are awake under spinal, TURP syndrome is recognized early.
- Excellent postoperative analgesia.

*Contraindications for Spinal Anesthesia*

- Patient refusal
- Infection at the site of spinal injection and systemic sepsis
- Raised intracranial pressure
- Coagulopathy
- Hypovolemia and shock.

The incidence of spinal headache (postdural puncture headache) is usually negligible due to thin needles and elderly patients. Foot-end elevation and immobilization of the patients to prevent spinal headache is not necessary in today's anesthetic practice.

## Epidural Analgesia

The indications and contraindications of epidural anesthesia are similar to the spinal anesthesia. It can be given alone or combined with spinal anesthesia. It is mainly preferred if the duration of surgery is uncertain or when postoperative analgesia is planned. This may be helpful, if there is a high probability of conversion to open prostatectomy.

## General Anesthesia

*Indications*

- Patient refusal for regional anesthesia
- Regional anesthesia is contraindicated
- Hemodynamic instability requiring inotropes
- Patients cannot lie flat
- When patients do not cooperate.

It is better to avoid GA in older patients, unless there are contraindications to regionals, as they do very well with regional anesthesia.

## POSITIONING-RELATED ISSUES

As patients undergoing TURP are in the elderly group, exquisite care should be taken during positioning for spinal anesthesia. Patients with arthritis and joint replacements need special attention while placing in lithotomy position to prevent dislocation. Adequate padding of the lateral aspect of knee should be done to prevent common peroneal nerve compression.

## COMPLICATIONS OF TRANSURETHRAL RESECTION OF PROSTATE

*Transurethral resection of prostate syndrome*—It is one of the morbid complications of TURP.

The fluid used as irrigant during resection is absorbed through opened blood vessels. The rough estimate is ≃15–30 mL/min and 900–1,800 mL/h. The amount absorbed depends on various factors. These solutions are moderately hypotonic and can be excessively absorbed. This can leading to TUR syndrome. The important characters of the various irrigants are shown in Table 5.2.

Transurethral resection of prostate syndrome is caused by absorption of irrigating fluid through ruptured sinuses and is associated with specific symptoms and signs.

Among the cardiovascular effects, the patient may have hypertension or hypotension, dysrhythmias (tachy/brady), congestive failure, pulmonary edema, hypoxemia of myocardial infarction.

*Glycine toxicity*: Very rare. Transient blindness, myocardial depression and delayed awakening can all occur due to glycine toxicity.

The CNS effects include agitation, confusion, headache, nausea, vomiting, seizures, coma, or visual disturbances (usually transient blindness). The CNS effects of TUR syndrome are contributed by not only hyponatremia, but also hypo-osmolality causing cerebral edema. Hyponatremia can cause CNS effects when levels go below 120 mEq/L and less than 115 mEq/L, produce ECG changes like QRS widening and ST elevation. Convulsions and coma can result from extreme hyponatremia less than 100 mEq/L. Severe hemolysis may occur due to hypo-osmolality.

Factors increasing the occurrence of TURP syndrome:

**Table 5.2:** Important characters of the various irrigants.

| Solution | Osmolality mOsm/kg | Advantages | Disadvantages |
|---|---|---|---|
| Distilled water | 0 | • Electrically inert<br>• Clear<br>• Inexpensive | • Hemolysis<br>• Hemoglobinuria<br>• Hyponatremia |
| Glycine (1.5%)<br>Glycine (1.2%) | 220 (iso)<br>175 (hypo) | Less chances for TURP syndrome | • Transient visual disturbance postoperative<br>• Hyperammonemia<br>• Hyperoxaluria |
| Normal saline (0.9%) | 308 (iso) | Less TURP syndrome | Conducts electricity. So cannot be used with diathermy |

- Large prostate gland (more than 45 g)
- Elderly age—more than 80 years
- Volume and type of irrigation fluid
- Height of the irrigation fluid
- Resection time (more than 60 min)
- Surgical experience
- Renal impairment.

## TREATMENT OF TRANSURETHRAL RESECTION OF PROSTATE SYNDROME

- Follow A, B and C—**a**irway, **b**reathing and **c**irculation
- Administer 100% oxygen
- Restrict fluids and administer loop diuretics like frusemide
- Whenever required awake patients or sedated patients may need to be sedated, intubated and ventilated
- Inform the surgeon to coagulate the bleeding points and terminate surgery as soon as possible
- Look for hypokalemia
- Rarely 3% NaCl may be used.

*Hypothermia*: Cold irrigation fluid and its absorption can cause hypothermia. Shivering may occur and this can increase the heart rate predisposing patients with IHD to myocardial ischemia and infarction. Warmed irrigation solution minimizes the occurrence of hypothermia.

*Bleeding and coagulopathy*: As there is a continuous irrigation of fluids for TURP it is difficult to estimate the blood loss. Some rough guidelines are given to assess the blood loss. Duration: 2-5 mL/min; size of the prostate—20-50 mL/g.

At the end of TURP procedure, lowering the legs from lithotomy position can cause severe hypotension due to reduction in venous return. Complications after TURP are hypothermia, hemorrhage, hypotension, septicemia and TURP syndrome which can be seen in the recovery room.

Newer technique for TURP like bipolar TURP allows normal saline to be used as the bladder irrigating fluid and minimizes chances of hyponatremia and hypo-osmolality and resultant TURP syndrome. But still, it is important to note that, it is not possible to prevent the possibility of volume overload. Lasers too minimize the blood loss and fluid absorption, especially if used for large glands.

## SPECIAL CONSIDERATIONS FOR TRANSURETHRAL RESECTION OF BLADDER TUMOR SURGERY

Transurethral resection of bladder tumor (TURBT) is a widely used surgical technique for both diagnosis and treatment of bladder cancer. It can be performed under spinal or general anesthesia depending on the site of the tumor.

TURBT cannot be carried out effectively due to sparing of obturator nerve, which courses on the lateral wall of bladder where it can get easily stimulated by the electrical current passed through the loop during resection with an intense involuntary response from adductors (adductor longus, brevis, magnus, gracilis) and external rotators (obturator externus) of hip. Adductor jerk or obturator reflex is associated with a serious injury such as vessel laceration with profuse bleeding, bladder wall tear or perforation, and even incomplete resection due to frequent distractions and interruptions to the operating surgeon.

Prophylaxis includes paralyzing the patients with muscle relaxants if under spinal or general anesthesia without muscle relaxants. A selective obturator nerve block especially under ultrasound guidance is the safest and most effective method to prevent obturator spasm.

## Obturator Nerve Block

Obturator reflex is not abolished by spinal anesthesia. Hence obturator nerve should be selectively blocked. Obturator block can be given with the help of an ultrasound or nerve stimulator or with anatomical landmarks.

## CONCLUSION

Transurethral resection of prostate is the gold standard surgery for BPH. The patients are elderly and hence every effort should be made to know their comorbidities. Generally spinal anesthesia is given for TURP. When GA is indicated adequate precautions should be taken. Positioning needs extra care in these patients. One should watch for TURP syndrome in these patients especially when the sinusoids are opened and the duration is more than 90 minutes. These patients should be monitored for complications in the postoperative period also. When TURBT is done one has to watch for excessive bleeding and obturator spasm. Avoid this spasm with obturator block or giving GA with muscle relaxants.

# Chapter 6

# Patient Preparation and Operation Theater Setup for Transurethral Resection

*M Anandan*

## INTRODUCTION

A common adage is "a good start is half job done".

A well prepared patient and setup is essential for the smooth course of surgery. A patient who is a candidate for the transurethral procedure is assessed for the medical fitness to undergo the procedure. This is discussed elsewhere in the book.

## PREOPERATIVE PREPARATION

Most of the patients undergoing transurethral resection of the prostate (TURP) are preceding medical management. Though α-blockers are used almost universally, 5α-reductase inhibitors (5ARIs) are used in select cases with large prostates. A recent meta-analysis in 2015 by Zhu et al. showed that the perioperative blood loss during TURP is decreased in those who are on 5ARIs. 2–4 weeks treatment is helpful.[1] In another randomized study by Arora et al. the authors reported decreased blood loss in those treated with 5ARIs.[2] The microvessel density in prostate has been found to be reduced with 5ARIs.[3] Though some studies report on the contrary, for a beginner, it is better to start 5ARIs once a patient is planned for TURP, so that the benefit, if at all present, is passed on to the patient.

The other common dilemma encountered is the patient presenting with acute retention. A recent review article published in 2015 strongly recommends *against* TURP immediately after acute urinary retention (AUR).[4] Many studies indicate that the complication rates and blood loss are high in those undergoing TURP immediately after retention. This might be due to the prostatic congestion due to retention. It is advisable to wait at least a week before TURP in those with retention of urine in the early part of the career.

All patients need a urine culture before proceeding for transurethral procedures. It is preferable to have a sterile urine prior to the procedure. But, in those with indwelling catheters, it can at least help in selecting the

# Patient Preparation and Operation Theater Setup for Transurethral Resection

appropriate antibiotics. The antibiotic prophylaxis depends on the antibiotic policy of the institute. If a previous culture report is available, corresponding antibiotics may be initiated at the time of induction. Else, a third generation cephalosporin is the preferred antibiotic in most institutions. Most guidelines suggest that a single dose is adequate for prophylaxis. But, it is preferable to continue at least till catheter removal, especially in case he needs irrigation, bladder wash, etc.

If the patient is habitually constipated, he needs proctoclysis enema on the day of surgery, to prevent the unwanted "mess" of defecation on the table after anesthesia or during the procedure. In those with normal bowel movement enema may be avoided. Moreover, some patients may need traction after the procedure with distended balloon. This can create a sensation of rectal fullness and the need to defecate. Prior rectal clearance helps in negating patient's apprehension of need to defecate in the immediate postoperative period.

## Patient Positioning

The proper patient positioning helps to provide a hassle free procedure for the surgeon and also prevents iatrogenic injuries to the patients.

The classical lithotomy position—right angles at the hip and knee with around 45° abduction at the hip is rarely necessary. A low lithotomy position with about 45° hip flexion and leg parallel to the floor is adequate. In the lithotomy rods with knee supports adequate padding should be provided to prevent common peroneal nerve injury (Figs. 6.1 and 6.2).

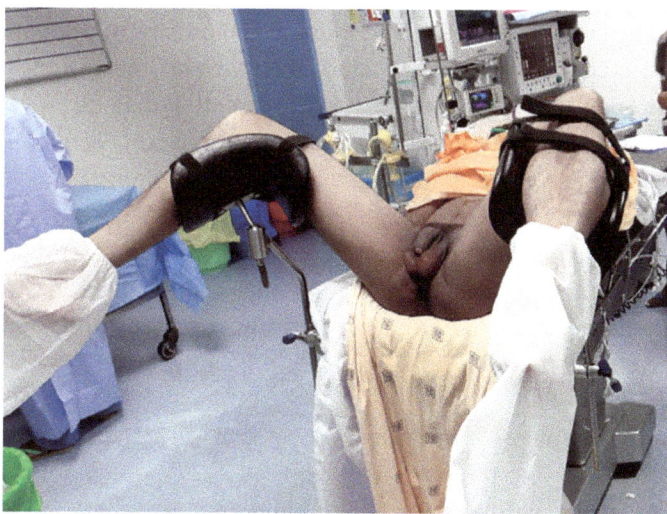

**Fig. 6.1:** Lithotomy position.

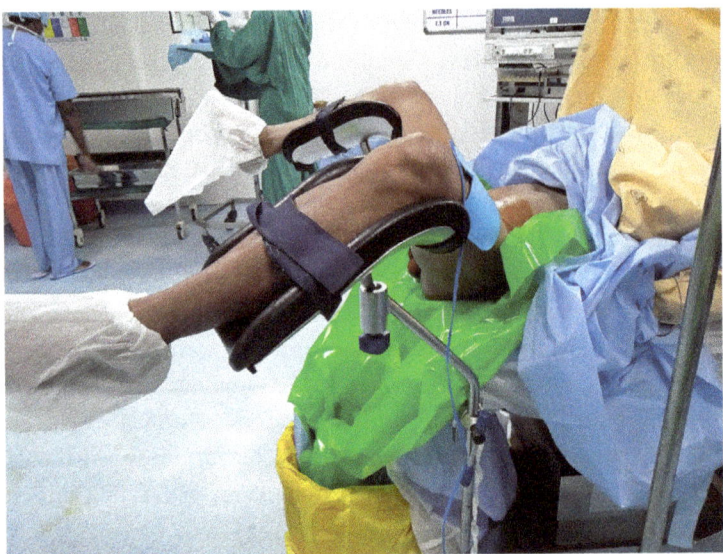

**Fig. 6.2:** Lithotomy position lateral view with probable position for securing the diathermy plate depicted.

The buttocks should be placed such that they are at the level of the edge of the table or projecting just beyond. This helps in tilting the resectoscope down without hindrance in those with high bladder neck or large median lobes.

The diathermy pads should be tightly secured to the torso and the patient positioning checked to identify any contact points with metallic structures of the table. The diathermy loads should be preferably placed under the gluteal muscles or secured to the thigh. Placing them in the upper part of the torso or arms should be avoided. This prevents the current taking the path "through" the heart and causing the remote possibility of arrhythmia. This is especially important in those with pacemakers (Fig. 6.2).

Genitalia, perineum, both thighs and lower abdomen below umbilicus should be prepared. Shaving just prior to the procedure is preferable. Sterile preparation of the same area is done as per the institute protocol. Preparation should be done till the umbilicus, since there may be a need to insert suprapubic catheter perioperatively, especially in large glands.

Instruments needed (Fig. 6.3):
- Cystoscope—30°.
- Cystoscope sheath with bridge—19 Fr to 22 Fr depending on surgeon preference.
- Resectoscope with both visual and blind obturator.

# Patient Preparation and Operation Theater Setup for Transurethral Resection

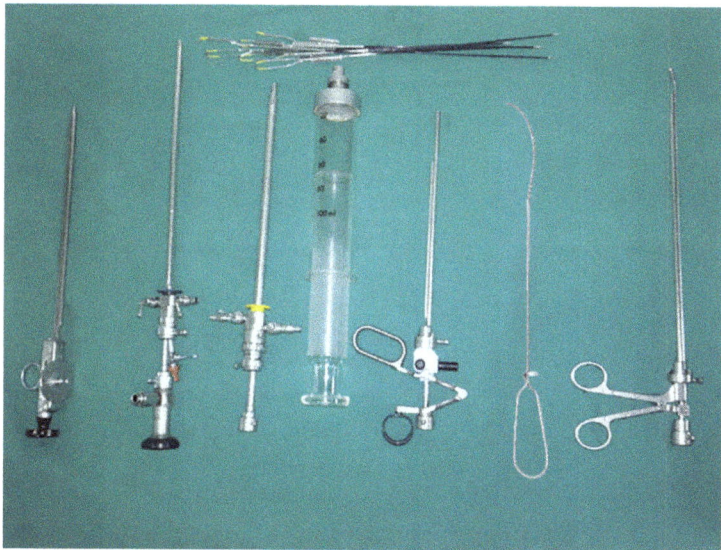

**Fig. 6.3:** Necessary instruments for transurethral resection.

- Irrigation fluid with connecting tubes.
- Camera set up.
- High frequency diathermy cables.
- Resection electrodes—loop (2), Collin's knife, and rollerball electrode.
- Chip evacuators—Ellick's evacuator/Toomey syringe/Alexander syringe.
- Strainer—to collect bits.
- Suprapubic trocar set—16 Fr, 18 Fr or 20 Fr.
- 20 Fr/22 Fr/24 Fr—3-way and 2-way Foley catheters.
- Foley catheter introducers.
- Otis urethrotome or Schashe's knife.
- Urethral dilators.

## Theater Setup for Transurethral Surgery

The operation theater should be adequately spacious for the instruments, monitors and the diathermy units. The probable set up for the theater personnel and the instruments is depicted in the Figure 6.3. The diathermy unit, if it is separate, can be placed toward the left side of the patient. The diathermy footswitch can be placed toward either foot of the surgeon depending on the comfort. Placing the diathermy machine on the side of the foot switch prevents entangling of the wires. The outlet tube can be placed into a bucket away from the Surgeon's legs. All the tubings should be secured to the drapes to prevent accidental slippage on the floor (Figs. 6.3 and 6.4).

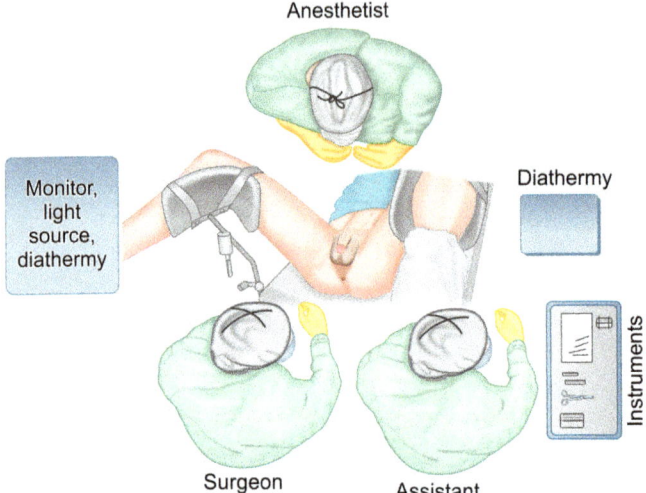

**Fig. 6.4:** Operation theater (OT) set up.

## REFERENCES

1. Zhu YP, Dai B, Zhang HL, et al. Impact of preoperative 5α-reductase inhibitors on perioperative blood loss in patients with benign prostatic hyperplasia: a meta-analysis of randomized controlled trials. BMC Urol. 2015;15:47.
2. Bansal A, Arora A. Transurethral resection of prostate and bleeding: A prospective randomized, double-blind placebo-controlled trial to see efficacy of short-term use of Finasteride and Dutasteride on operative blood loss and prostatic microvessel density. J Endourol. 2017;31:910-7.
3. Sugie S, Mukai S, Tsukino H, et al. Effect of dutasteride on microvessel density in benign prostatic hyperplasia. In Vivo. 2014;28:355-9.
4. Yoon PD, Chalasani V, Woo HH. Systematic review and meta-analysis on management of acute urinary retention. Prostate Cancer Prostatic Dis. 2015;18:297-302.

# Chapter 7

# Basics of Transurethral Resection

*M Anandan*

## INTRODUCTION

The technique of transurethral resection is akin to removing a tumor piecemeal in open/laparoscopic surgery. We need to remove the tumor, control the bleeding, and stop when the margin (capsule) is reached.

Before embarking on resection, basic cystoscopy is a must. This needs to be done with a 20 or 21 Fr sheath. This helps in the preliminary assessment of the anterior urethra, prostate gland, and the bladder before inserting the larger 26 Fr rotating sheath (Fig. 7.1)

The resectoscope sheath can be inserted using the blind obturator or "under vision" with the help of Schmidt's obturator. In cases with large median lobes, as defined by preliminary cystoscopy, using Schmidt's obturator prevents injury and subtrigonal perforation. Generous use of lubricant jelly is advisable for smooth insertion of the resectoscope sheath.

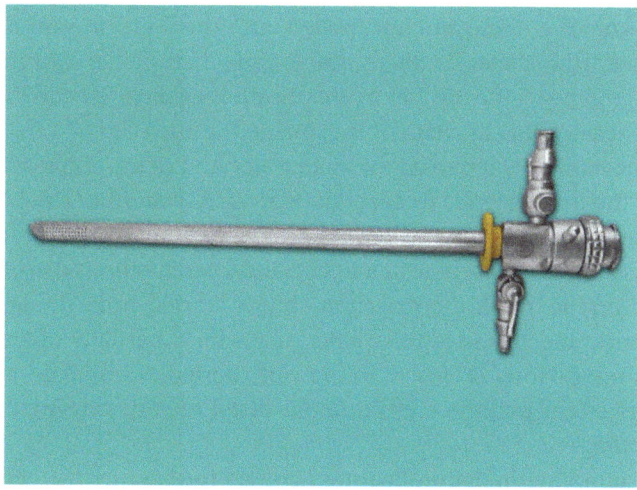

**Fig. 7.1:** 26 Fr rotating sheath.

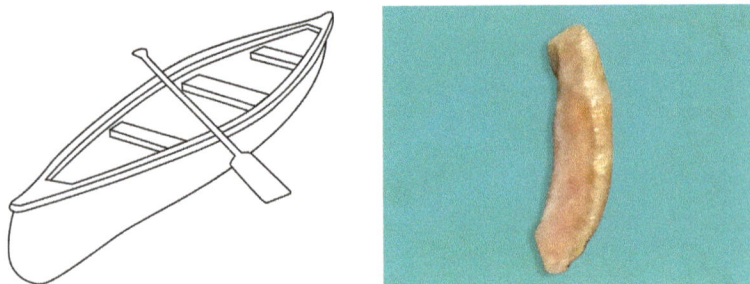

**Fig. 7.2:** Boat (canoe) shaped chips.

In those with narrow meatus, it can be dilated with metal dilators, or ventral meatotomy can be done for facilitating sheath insertion. In those with narrow urethra, Otis urethrotomy is helpful in widening it and prevents later development of strictures. Few authors suggest using Otis urethrotomy in all cases prior to resection. In some patients, smaller sheaths—24 Fr, without continuous flow can be used.

The landmarks must be identified prior to transurethral resection. Verumontanum (veru) and ureteric orifices need to be positively identified prior to the start of resection. Since the distal limit of resection is the veru, the sheath beak should be stationed at the level of veru and the resection should be done with the movement of loop alone (without movement of the sheath)—at least in the initial part of training. This prevents inadvertent extension of resection beyond veru.

The sheath beak is placed at the level of the veru and the loop is extended till the bladder neck or just proximal to it. The classical description of a "good" resection chip is of the boat or blunt trapezoid shape (Fig. 7.2). This shape will be obtained with the movement of the loop so that the chip is "cut out" from the tissue and not "pulled out". The initial inward movement is angulated, (the sheath is tilted), the loop is then pulled into the sheath, when the loop nears the insulation, the sheath is again tilted and loop pulled out of the tissue. This movement is explained in the (Figs. 7.3 to 7.5).

This movement is repeated multiple times and many chips of tissue are resected. The loop extends to a length of around 3 cm from the beak of the sheath. Hence, for glands smaller than this length, movement of sheath is not necessary. But, in those with longer glands, two methods can be applied.

In the first method, the resection chip is started from the level of the bladder neck and the sheath is pulled out with a partially open loop, till the veru and the loop is closed. In the early period of training, rather such maneuvers might pull the sheath too far distal to veru causing damage to the sphincter.

In the other method, the sheath is inserted further proximal to the veru, and the loop is extended fully till the bladder neck. The resection is done for

## Basics of Transurethral Resection

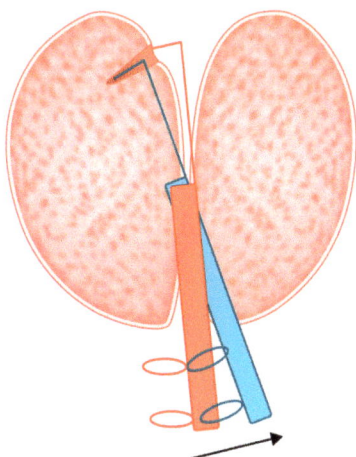

**Fig. 7.3:** Initial movement of sheath to insert loop into the prostate parenchyma.

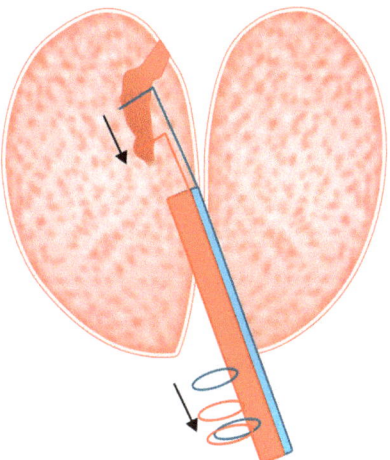

**Fig. 7.4:** Chip being resected from the prostate.

the proximal part of the prostate. Then the sheath is moved distally till the veru and then the distal part of the prostate is resected. With this technique, the possibility of moving the sheath beyond the veru and damaging the sphincter is negated.

The depth of penetration of the loop is 3-4 mm. Complete immersion of the loop into the tissue helps in procuring thicker resection chips, especially in large glands and helps to reduce the operation time. The end of the loop can be bent inward so that the chip is cut with minimal movement of the sheath. It is better to avoid the loop coming too close to the scope to prevent thermal damage to the lens. The loop should be always under vision and

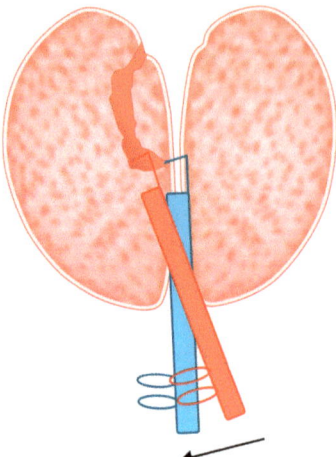

**Fig. 7.5:** Sheath is tilted inward so that the loop moves from the prostate parenchyma, toward the urethra to complete the resection of chip.

should stop 1 mm before the beak and the chip should be resected at the level. In some instances, the distal cut of the chip can be affected with the loop engaging with the insulation of the sheath.

Though the loop is of uniform thickness throughout, with the resection in progress, the central part gets thinned out faster than the lateral parts. The thinner part, which concentrates the current more, is helpful for cutting and the lateral parts can be used for coagulation.

## CONTROL OF BLEEDING

The most important part of the resection is control of bleeding. The simplest technique is to place the loop directly over the bleeder and coagulating it. If possible the lateral 'limbs' of the loop can be used for coagulation. The thinner loop might, in some instances, might plough through the gland causing more bleed. Direct "point coagulation" is better than sweeping movement over the bleeder (Figs. 7.6A and B).

In larger bleeds or venous bleeds, which do not get controlled with direct coagulation, loop can be applied proximal to the bleeding point and the feeding vessel can be coagulated. The other technique is to compress the walls of the vessel while applying the coagulation current (Fig. 7.7).

In some instances, the field is reddish with difficulty in identifying the bleeder. In such cases, the scope is withdrawn toward the veru and the probable quadrant of the bleeder can be identified. Else, the scope is pushed till the bladder neck and gradually withdrawn. Due to the tamponade effect of the sheath, the field improves a little and the scope is withdrawn viewing each sextant. It is better to keep the loop slightly open so that the bleeder, if identified, is coagulated at once.

# Basics of Transurethral Resection

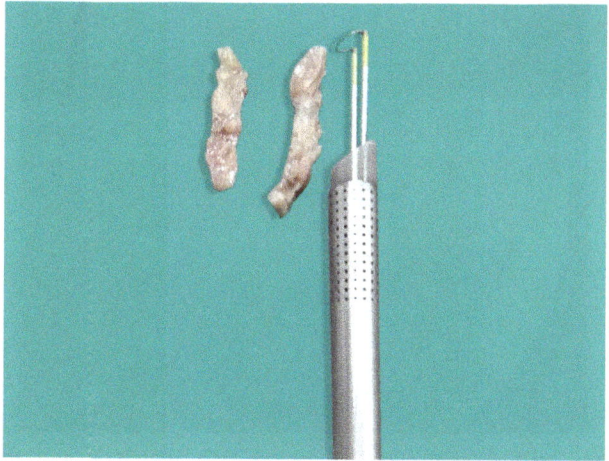

Prostate chips of exposed loop length.

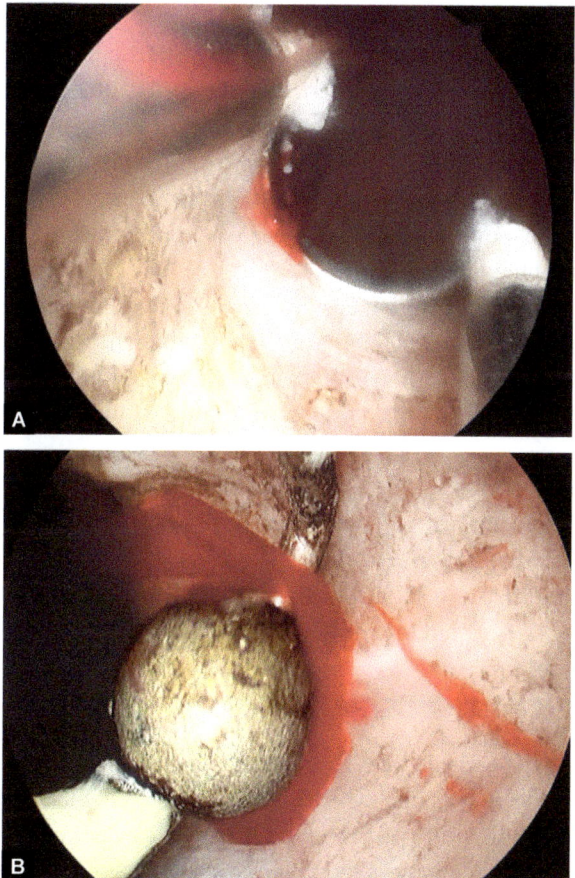

**Figs. 7.6A and B:** Arterial bleeder controlled by direct application of diathermy—(A) Loop; or (B) Ball can be used.

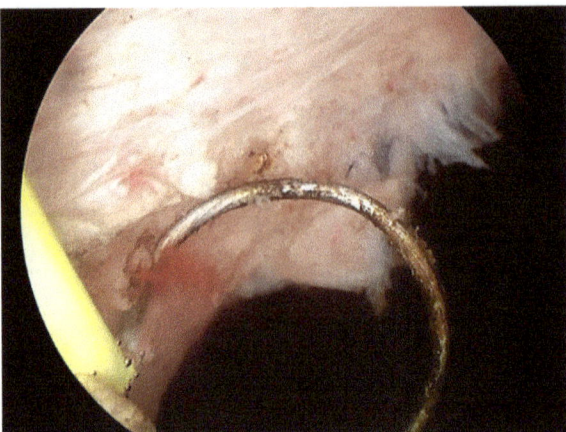

**Fig. 7.7:** Large bleeder controlled by compression with loop and application of coagulation current.

If the bleeding is suspected to be form a particular quadrant, but if a thorough examination is futile in identifying the bleeder, it could be a ricochet bleeding from the opposite wall. In many instances the bleeding from the anterior wall due to the abrasion from the sheath is the culprit. In case where the bleeder is directly sputing on to the scope, slightly forward or backward movement to change in the orientation of the scope will help to identify the bleeder.

In those instances, where it is still difficult to find the bleeder, the inflow pressure can be increased by increasing the height of the irrigant and usually the bleeder is identified. This has to be done with caution, since open sinus with high pressure irrigation can cause increased intravasation and TUR syndrome.

In the final stages, if there is some diffuse ooze and definite is not identified, decreasing the inflow will make the bleeder show up and it can be tackled. Finally, ball electrode can be used to "roll over" the prostatic capsule to cauterize the small bleeders. Ball electrode can also be used to tackle slightly larger bleeders not controlled with loop.

## DIFFERENTIATION OF GLAND AND CAPSULE

Differentiating the capsule from the gland is essential in avoiding perforation. The glandular tissue gets cut easily with cutting current, like cutting through soap. The off-white color of the gland changes to brown char in case of glandular tissue. The capsule is identified by the characteristic pearly white or pinkish color, without any brownish discoloration on application of current.

## Basics of Transurethral Resection

The other finding is that the capsule moves outward with the application of pressure loop, whereas glandular tissue is not pliable. Prominent venous sinuses may be seen through the capsule. Direct application of diathermy to the capsule will cause capsular contraction. This is also one of the identifying features. Resecting beyond the capsule leads to perforation (Figs. 7.4 to 7.6)

The fine crisscrossing fibers are also identified in the capsule. Prominent fibers with minimal cobweb indicate impending perforation and identification of fat in the field shows means complete perforation (Figs. 7.8 to 7.14).

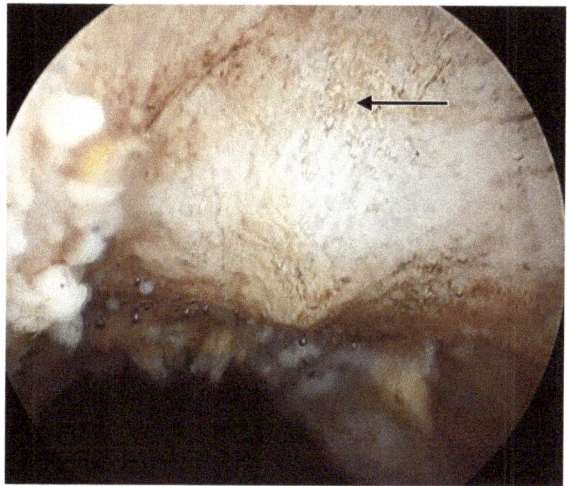

**Fig. 7.8:** Yellowish brown appearance of adenoma (arrow).

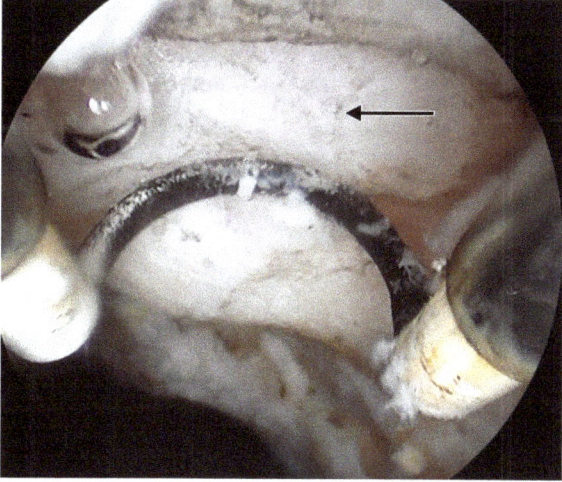

**Fig. 7.9:** Fine pearly white glistening capsule (arrow).

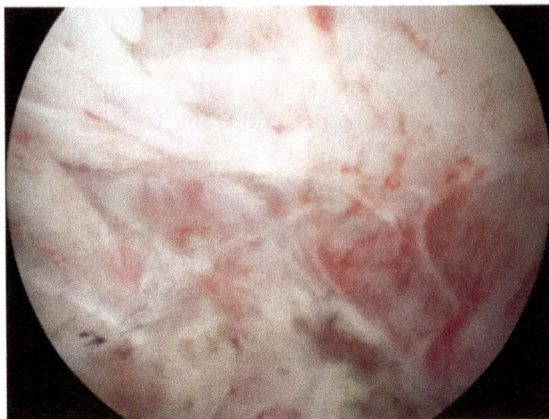

**Fig. 7.10:** Deeper capsular resection—impending perforation—thick crisscross fibers seen.

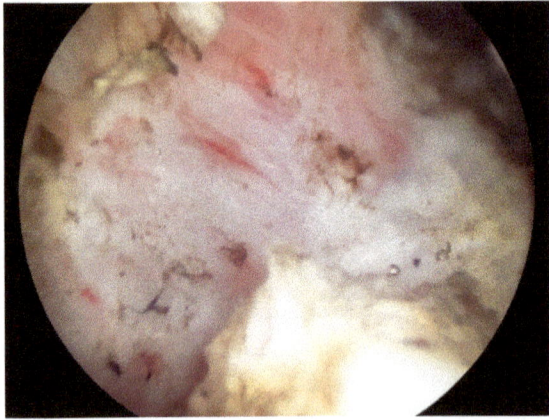

**Fig. 7.11:** Superficial layer of capsule—fine parallel fibers.

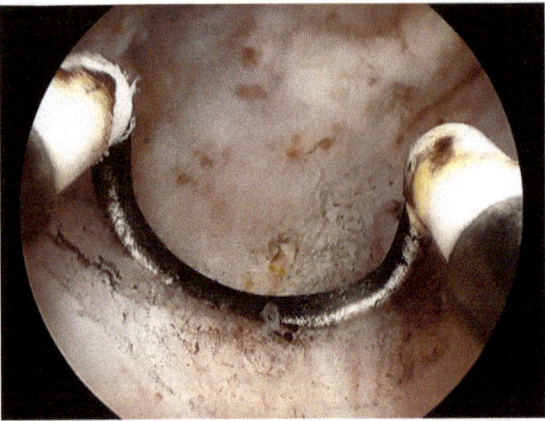

**Fig. 7.12:** Prostatic calcification at the level of capsule.

# Basics of Transurethral Resection

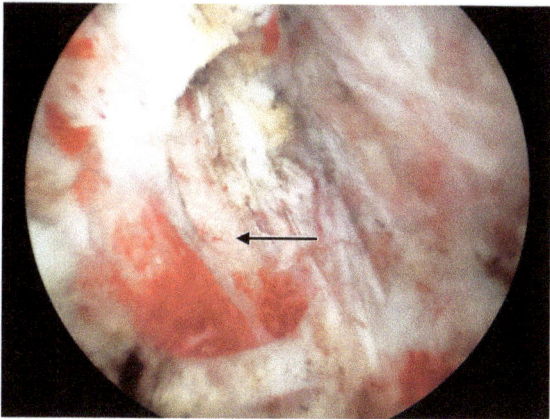

**Fig. 7.13:** Capsular perforation with fat exposed (arrow).

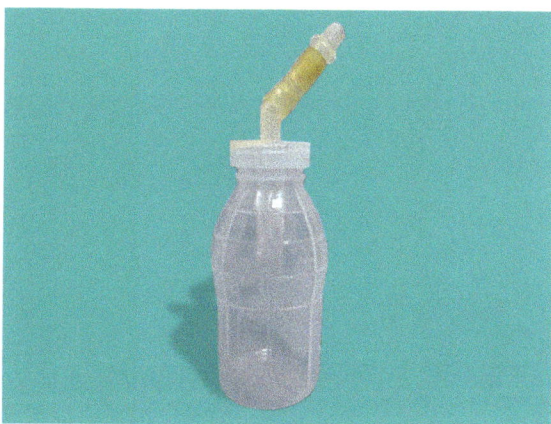

**Fig. 7.14:** Modified Ellick's evacuator.

## REMOVAL OF RESECTED CHIPS

The evacuators are used for removal of resected prostate chips. Ellick's evacuator, Toomey's syringe, Alexander's syringe is the commonly used evacuators. The classical Ellick's evacuator consisted of a dumbbell-shaped glass bottle with an offset tube channel and bulb at the end. It is initially filled with saline or water *without air bubbles* and the tube channel is connected to the sheath end. Activation of the bulb removes the chips by passive suction effect. The heavy chips settle down in the lower part of the dumbbell. The bulb should be activated slowly to give time for the chips to settle down. Air bubbles create foam hampering the evacuation of chips.

One simple trick is to angulate the sheath toward the base of the bladder while activating the balloon to displace the prostatic chips. Then the sheath

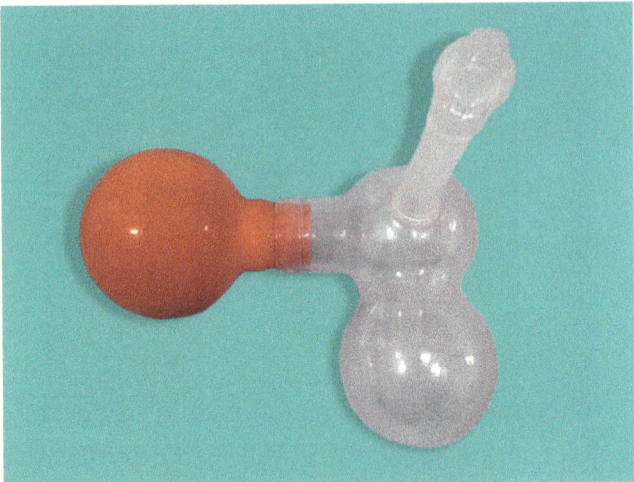

**Fig. 7.15:** Classical Ellick's evacuator.

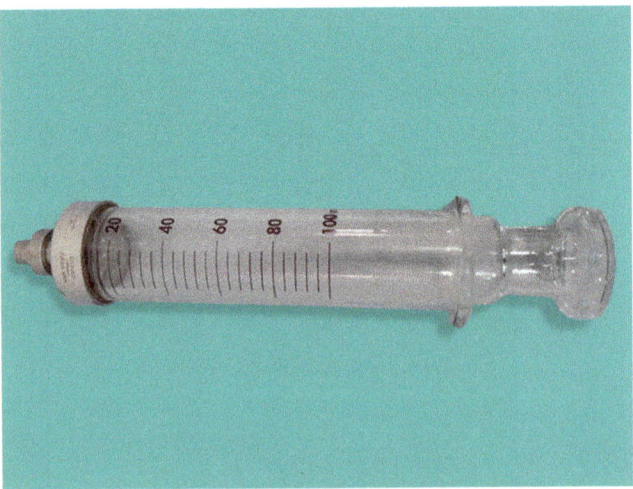

**Fig. 7.16:** Toomey syringe.

is straightened to remove the floating bits during the passive suctioning effect.

The Toomey syringe and Alexander syringe can be used either prefilled, or can be filled with the irrigation fluid after attaching them to the sheath. Incomplete return of the instilled fluid could be due to the bladder mucosa or large prostate bit impinging into the sheath tip. A little manipulation of the resectoscope or flushing with more fluid with help dislodge them (Figs. 7.15 to 7.16).

# Chapter 8

# Transurethral Monopolar Resection of the Prostate

*Ganesh Gopalakrishnan*

## HISTORY

The cornerstone of monopolar resection has to be the diathermy unit. The Egyptians are considered to be among the first to use cautery to treat patient conditions. Cautery is mentioned as a treatment to control hemorrhage in Ebers Papyrus, believed to be written around 1500 BC. The use of cautery during the 16th century declined due to another preferred modality-ligature used to control bleeding and was introduced by Ambroise Paré. Resurgence in the field of electrosurgery was due to the work of William Gilbert who was recognized as the father of electrotherapy. More light has been thrown on this field following the work of Benjamin Franklin, Luigi Galvani, and Michael Faraday.

Physicists had known that a spark between two electrodes alternates in direction and spark gaps were used in the 1890s to produce alternating currents with a frequency of 100,00/sec.

Spark gap oscillations are irregular and currents delivered by spark gaps machines are said to be damped. Damped currents coagulate tissue. The cutting instrument was a pointed electrode that concentrated current in a small volume of tissue and a large indifferent electrode.

Reinhold Wappler made the electrical apparatus for spark gap cautery and in 1908 Edwin Beer a New York genitourinary surgeon asked Wappler if this technology would be useful in urology. The cautery had to work under water in the urinary bladder. Wappler said that it would not work but Beer found that it did and used it to treat warts submerged in water.

He then introduced a cystoscope with an insulated wire in an 81-year-old woman with a bladder tumor and was able to cauterize it by application of the bare end of the wire against the tumor and was able to destroy it in seconds. He went onto suggest that it might be useful in transurethral prostatectomy. His suggestion was taken up by Stevens of Bellevue Hospital in New York in 1913 and described how he relived prostatic obstruction by cauterizing in 3 minutes. Bugbee also reported results on 14 patients using a bare end of an insulated copper wire through an 18 Fr cystoscope.

In 1920 vacuum tubes were substituted for spark gaps. In 1926 Maximilian Stern of New York described the use of low-voltage radiofrequency current to cut slivers of prostatic tissue with a 0.5 cm ring of tungsten wire drawn through his resectoscope.

Joseph McCarthy substituted the Stern metal sheath with Bakelite with the help of Frederick Wappler. They attached an incandescent light at the end of a straight cystoscope and the U-shaped bit of wire by a rack and pinion movement within the sheath of the resectoscope.

This design of the Stern-McCarthy resectoscope was used for many years by many genitourinary surgeons and much before Harvey Cushing described his use of electrosurgery in removal of intracranial tumors.

It was Cushing at a World Congress who introduced William Bovie to explain to the audience the nuances of electrocautery. Bovie constructed a vacuum tube generator to deliver both cutting and coagulating current. The assistant would choose either by a turn of a switch. Nesbit in 1931, ordered a resectoscope and an electrical generator from Liebel-Flarsheim company in Cincinnati. He practiced cutting of pieces of beef the previous night and the next day proceeded to complete a closed transurethral resection of the prostate (TURP).

Nesbit initially used the rack and pinion system of the resectoscope but later modified it to a single handed instrument with a spring mechanism to move the loop.

He also used a 33 Fr sheath and when this was too large to be inserted into the urethra he made a button-hole urethrotomy in the bulbar urethra to insert the instrument. This technique may need to be followed albeit rarely today if one encounters such a situation. Wappler later made for him smaller sheaths of 24 Fr and 26 Fr. These were the earliest prototypes of the resectoscope which are used today. The basic fundamental design is still the same but were more refined and sleeker in appearance.

The modern diathermy units have abandoned the old spark gap technology and moved into solid state components. These machines are sleeker, easily portable, robust, and able to deliver high wattage energy to both resect and vaporize prostatic tissue.

## TRANSURETHRAL INCISION AND RESECTION OF THE PROSTATE

There are essentially two procedures that are possible using monopolar energy to treat prostatic obstruction. The first is transurethral incision of the prostate (TUIP) popularized by Orandi.[1] A simple and effective procedure which unfortunately has fallen off the radar and needs to be revived. The second is the conventional TURP (Figs. 8.1 to 8.5). In spite of the plethora of techniques for treating prostatic problems, this method still stands as

# Transurethral Monopolar Resection of the Prostate

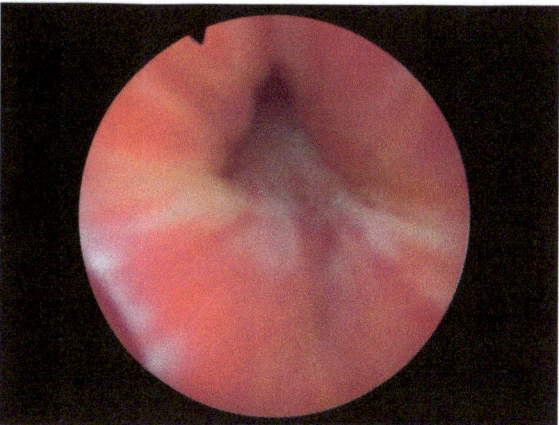

**Fig. 8.1:** Appearance of distal sphincter.

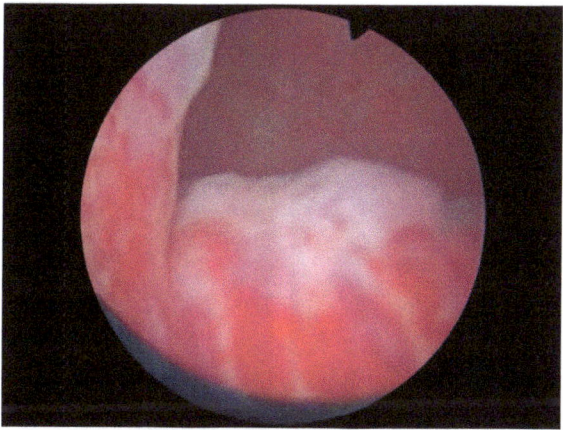

**Fig. 8.2:** Small median lobe.

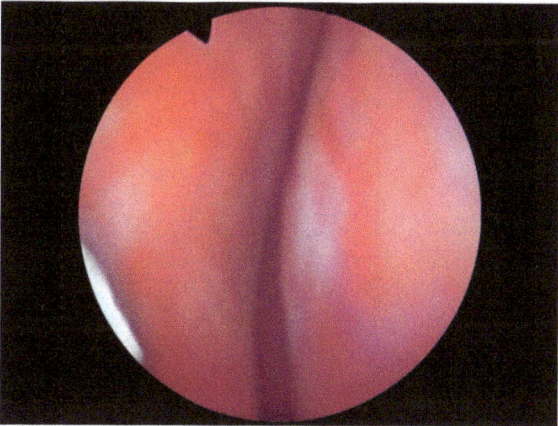

**Fig. 8.3:** Occlusive lateral lobe.

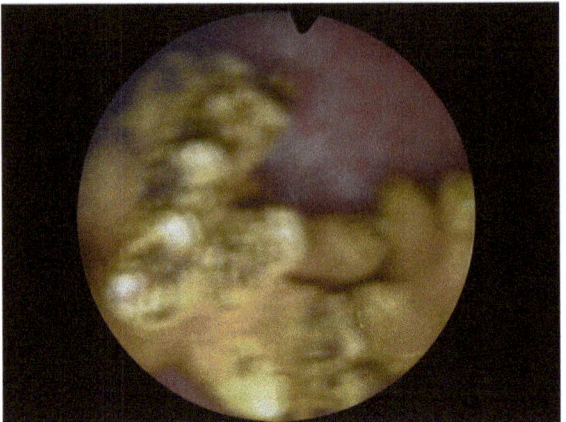

**Fig. 8.4:** Large bladder jackstone calculus.

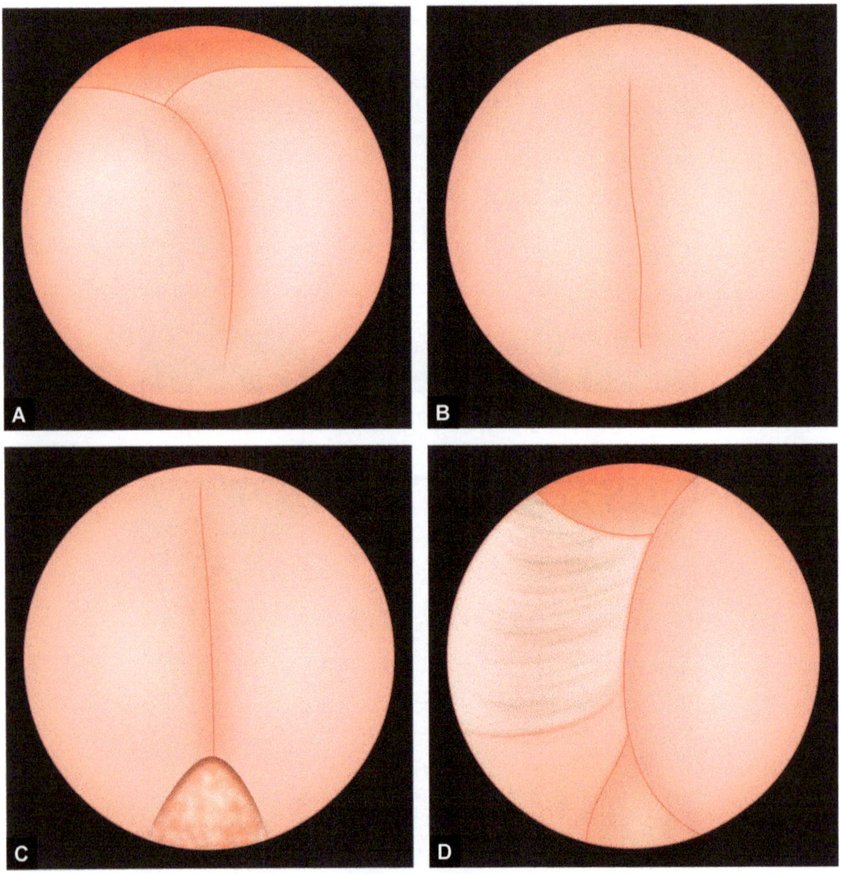

**Figs. 8.5A to D**

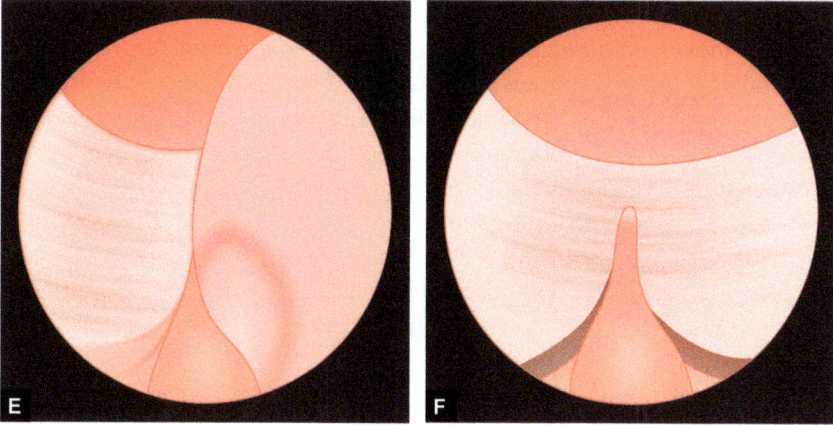

**Figs. 8.5E and F**

**Figs. 8.5A to F:** (A) A small view of the bladder cavity and the presence of two large lateral lobes; (B) Presence of the lateral lobes and the very markedly narrowed urethra; (C) Lateral lobes and the verumontanum; (D) Partial removal of the right lobe; (E) Complete removal of the right lobe; and (F) Complete removal of both lobes. The verumontanum is intact.

the most popular and used by the vast majority of urologists globally. It is cheap, effective and has stood the challenge against the many minimally invasive techniques for treating prostatic obstruction of a benign nature. It is a procedure which separated the general surgeons from the urologists and certainly the men from the boys. Its problem is a steep learning curve and takes time to master. In spite of this, seasoned resectionists can certainly get themselves into difficulty especially when faced with large glands for resection.

## Transurethral Incision of the Prostate

Transurethral incision of the prostate has been underutilized for treatment of bladder outflow obstruction. Commonly it is used for young men, some of whom may be unmarried, when they have urodynamically proven bladder outflow obstruction with bilateral upper tract obstruction or even elevated serum creatinine. These men have no endoscopic evidence of prostate occlusion and hence it is reasonable to classically carry out a bladder neck incision (BNI). While this is probably sufficient to just incise the bladder neck region alone, it is more common to incise the entire length of the prostatic urethra from just inside the bladder neck up to the verumontanum. The risk of retrograde ejaculation which is 100% with a formal TURP is significantly lower with bilateral neck incision and even more lower with a single incision (10%).[2] Single incision of the bladder neck is adequate to achieve efficient voiding and improvement in renal parameters.

Of all the prostatectomies performed in France in 1992, only 4% were done by TUIP. In 1806, Sir William Blizard performed the first BNI through a perineal urethrotomy. It gained some popularity but when the concept of prostatectomy was introduced, its use began to wane. When Stern introduced the resectoscope in 1926, the emphasis turned to prostatic resection.

It was Keitzer in 1961, who reintroduced this procedure. In 1973, Orandi[1] published an article on 40 patients who had undergone this procedure. In the same year Turner Warwick[3] published his series on BNI and slowly it became an accepted technique.

The primary indication for TUIP with or without BNI is symptomatic bladder outlet obstruction (BOO) in conjunction with benign prostatic hyperplasia (BPH). The indication for TUIP is actually the same as for TURP, the one difference being the size of the prostate. TUIP has proved to be efficient in prostate with smaller volumes around 30 mL (30 g). In Orandi's original article he estimated prostate size by cystoscopy.

It is also a useful treatment modality for younger patients in whom preservation of retrograde ejaculation is crucial. The more recent technique of prostatic incision has the same indications. One of the drawbacks of the procedure is failure to get tissue for histology. Of course that would not make a difference in the older person because of PSA testing and evaluation using multiparametric MRI.

The Figure 8.6 shows diagrammatically the lines of incision for both a selective BNI and TUIP.

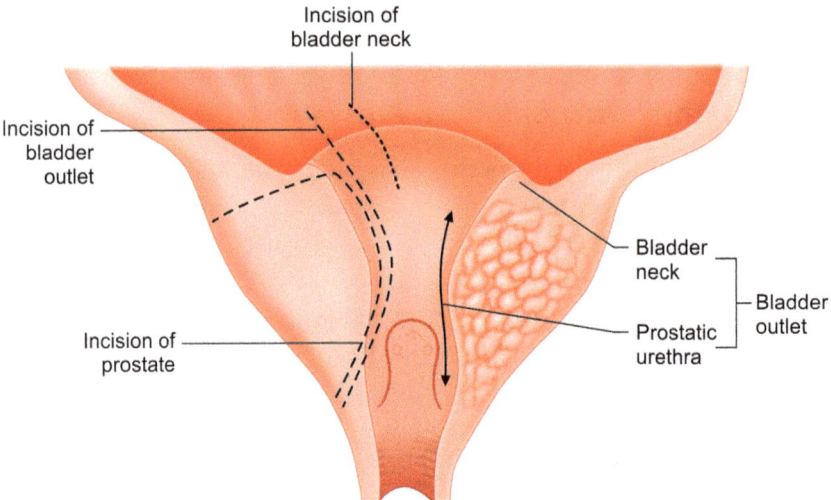

**Fig. 8.6:** Bladder neck incision and transurethral incision of the prostate.

## Transurethral Resection of the Prostate (Figs. 8.7 to 8.10)

Transurethral resection of the prostate was introduced in the early 1930s by pioneers whose names have been etched in urological history—Davis, Alcock, Nesbit, Stern, McCarthy, and Barnes. Needless to say that this procedure took its roots in the USA and came much later across the Atlantic to the UK brought by stalwarts like John Blandy. In India, it was Roger Barnes, from Loma Linda in the USA who while on a sabbatical to the Christian Medical College, Vellore in the mid-60s taught this technique to Prof. HS Bhat—the father of modern urology in India. Many other senior urologists whose names include Mansingh, Bapna, and Gangwal had learnt this technique while overseas and brought it back with them on their return.

Transurethral resection of the prostate is a difficult operation to master and the earlier sceptics would ridicule it as an operation that would create a "button-hole" in the prostate. In 1989, in a survey conducted by the AUA, 70% of the responders felt that there needed to be a minimum of 75 resections done during the residency to achieve adequate proficiency in the art. Today with the advent of drugs and other minimally invasive techniques, the citadel on which TURP was crowned as the "gold standard" is being shaken.

Today, there have been significant advances in the field of optics, electrosurgery and imaging that has enabled TURP to be learnt better and maybe marginally easier. The excellent quality of optics namely the Hopkins rod-lens system, the ergonomic resectoscope design, the three-chip camera and the high quality diathermy units enable residents to watch the procedure and then be instructed with hands on training with the consultant observing close at hand ready to take over in the event of any misadventure. Additionally, surgery and endoscopic surgery in particular has taken a leaf out of the aviation industry and TURP simulators are available which can also be incorporated into resident training programs and enable better hand—eye and foot coordination.

In the initial days of learning, it is advisable to start with smaller glands and then slowly progress with time and gaining confidence to tackle larger glands.

How much of the prostate should be resected; how much time can be allowed to do the procedure safely; can I resect the prostate in two sittings and is there a concept of hemi-resection of the prostate.

These are often asked questions by residents.

It is ideal that the entire adenoma be resected and up to the surgical capsule all around. However, it is well accepted that this may not be the case overall and in some area small amounts of prostatic tissue is left behind. This does appear to affect the overall outcome both in the short and in the

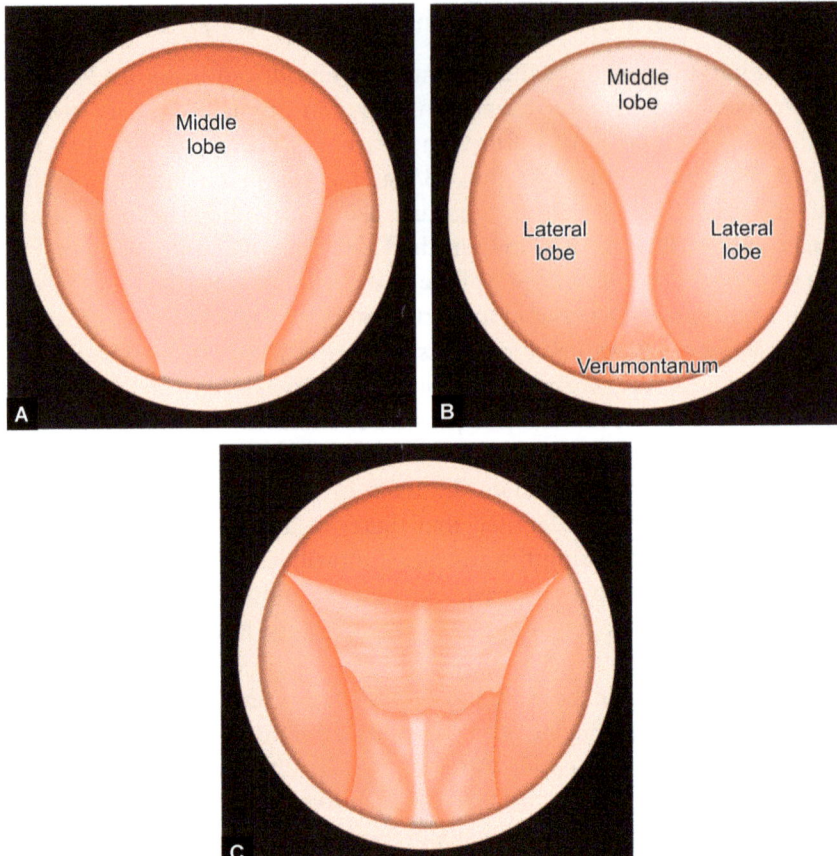

**Figs. 8.7A to C:** (A) Presence of a middle lobe; (B) View showing the lateral lobes, the middle lobe, and the verumontanum; and (C) Beginning resection of the middle lobe.

long term in the vast majority of patients. It is of interest to note that in a cooperative study of 3855 TURPs by Mebust,[4] 80% resections yielded 30 g or less of tissue. This would indicate that in majority of cases it is important for the surgeon to determine preoperatively the volume of the prostate and decide if it is within his/her ability to resect the gland. Attempting a TURP on a large gland by an inexperienced resectionist is not sound judgment and could result invariably in incomplete resection, bleeding, and other complications.

To resect a large gland will naturally take time. The average speed of resection has been quoted as 1 g of tissue or more per minute for an experienced resectionist. For a beginner it will be less. Irrespective of the above, the time duration spent for the resection should at best not exceed 60-90 minutes. Nevertheless, most experienced resectionists would say that they have gone up to 120 minutes in the odd case and the patient has not come to any harm. Increasing the time spent for resection will increase the absorption of fluid

# Transurethral Monopolar Resection of the Prostate

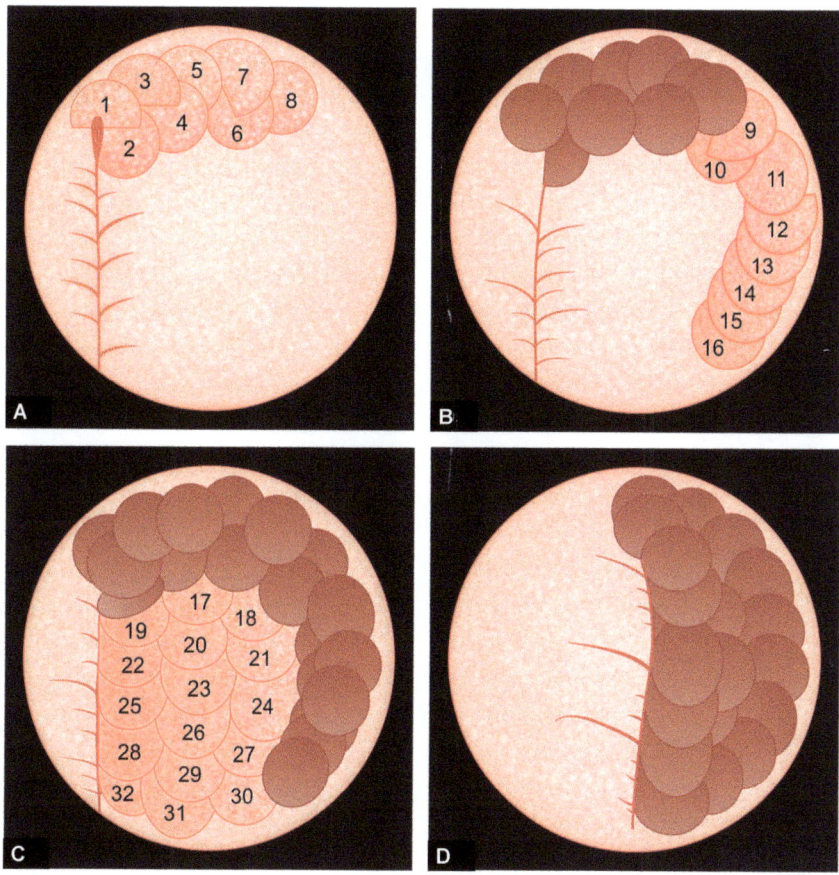

**Figs. 8.8A to D:** Resection of left lateral lobe. (A) Resection at 12o'clock; (B) Resection continues clockwise staying close to capsule; (C) This makes the medial mass of prostate avascular alloweing rapid resection; (D) Completed left lobe resection.

and result in fluid overload. In the earlier days, when water was the irrigant solution being used for TURP, transurethral resection (TUR) syndrome with acute tubular necrosis and hemolysis was a consequence every urologist was afraid of as the mortality was very high. Today with the use of iso-osmotic solutions this risk has considerably diminished.

Today's resectoscopes have improved in design and the entry of the continuous flow resectoscope has allowed for longer resection times. The use of the Reuter cannula in the bladder by some urologists has also helped. Both these techniques serve to keep the intravesical pressure low during the procedure and thereby reducing the risk of fluid absorption.

The old adage "there are many ways to skin a cat" may not be applicable to TURP. There are three well described techniques for resection—(1) Nesbit, (2) Alcocks, and (3) Barnes and it is advisable to stick to a standard plan of

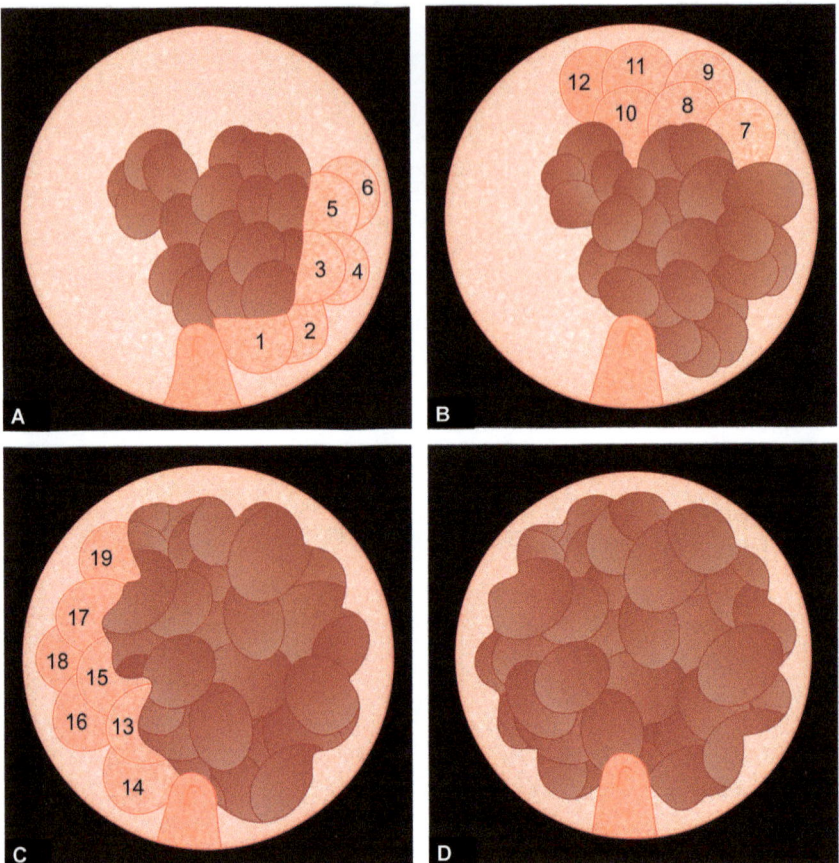

**Figs. 8.9A to D:** Resection of the apex. (A) Residual adenoma surrounds verumontanum; (B) Continuing resection counter clockwise; (C) Resection of right side at apex and continuing clockwise; (D) Apical resection is complete.

resection not only in the earlier part of the learning but also later as one gains competence and confidence. It is very poor judgment if one jumps from one section of the prostate to another while doing the procedure. Complete one lobe at a time and achieve hemostasis before proceeding to the next. If during the process one exceeds the safe time limit, the resection can be stopped and the patient brought back in 48 hours to complete the procedure. Most patients will void quite satisfactorily even after a one lobe resection.[5]

### Technique of Transurethral Resection of the Prostate

While it is not advisable to dictate to the anesthetist as to the type of anesthesia for a TURP, by and large most TURPs are done under spinal analgesia. The spinal anesthetic agents used today provide a maximum

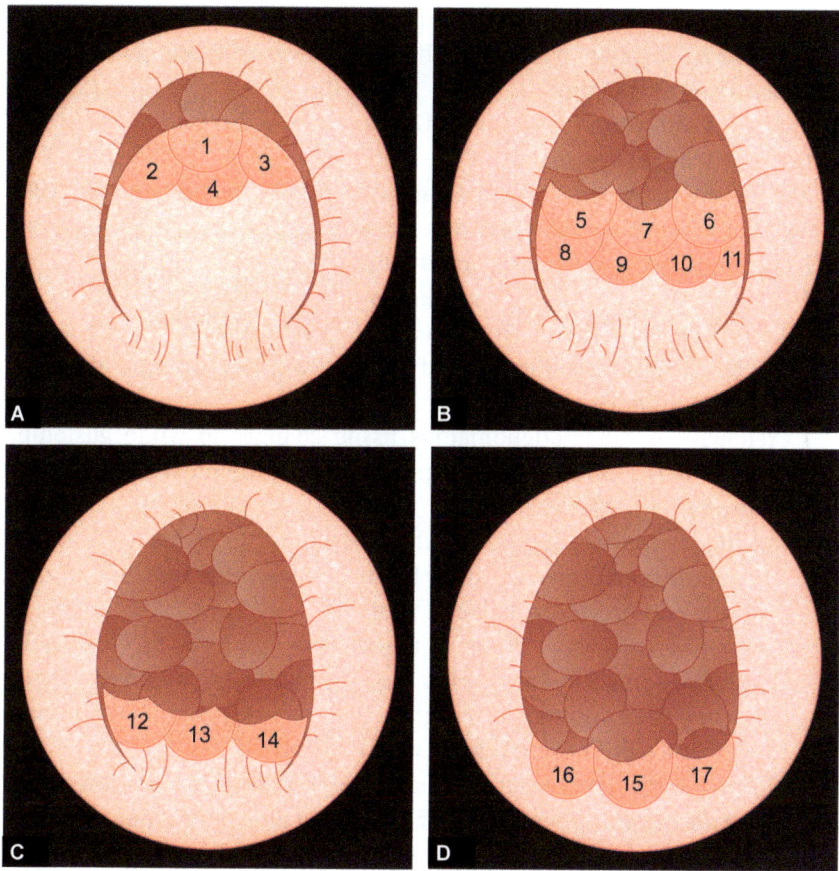

**Figs. 8.10A to D:** Resection of intravesical median lobe. (A to C) Location and sequence of cuts of middle lobe during resection; (D) Resection of the base of the middle lobe.

of 2 hours of resection time and sometimes even more. This is adequate time for a seasoned resectionist to even complete a larger gland; while it is time enough for a beginner to learn the skills without compromising the situation. In studies evaluating the effect of anesthesia on blood loss, complications, and operative mortality, McGowan[6] and Nielsen[7] found no substantial difference between regional and general anesthesia.

Prior to embarking on a TURP, it is important for the surgeon to make sure that his instruments are ready, sterile, in good working condition. This is akin to an airline pilot who does the preflight checks after each landing and take off. The diathermy, the camera, irrigant fluid, and endoscopic equipment consisting of the cystoscope, urethral bougies, Otis urethrotome, continuous flow resectoscope with a wide range of loops, and the telescope.

Transurethral resection of the prostate is a solo effort and you cannot blame anyone if things go wrong. There are however a few points worth reemphasizing at this time:
- There is a safety time limit for a TURP and this is dictated by the size of the gland, its vascularity and the experience of the resectionist.
- The verumontanum is the most constant and useful landmark in TURP.
- Adenomatous tissue can extend beyond the verumontanum and should be resected without jeopardizing the distal sphincter.
- Under-resection is always better than over resection.
- While resecting, it is important to know what the capsule looks like so that it is not breached. The fibers of the surgical capsule can be identified by a few landmarks:
  - Yellowish nodular adenomatous tissue changes to white glistening surface of the compressed peripheral zone of the prostate or surgical capsule.
  - Another important landmark which identifies the surgical capsule is the presence of prostatic calculi located between the transitional zone and the compressed peripheral zone.
  - The white transverse fibers of the bladder neck are the first to be identified sometimes as soon as the first loop length of the prostate is resected. It is important to recognize this and not breach this landmark as it will result in undermining of the trigone.
- Following completion of the resection especially in larger glands the bladder neck is wide open. However, in some smaller fibrous and moderate size glands, the bladder neck looks still narrowed endoscopically. In such cases an additional bladder neck incision[8] is useful and helps prevent bladder neck contracture.

### Training in Transurethral Resection of the Prostate

There are many ways to learn TURP. Initially one needs to observe the mentor on the monitor. The next step is to practice on the simulator. Simulators are expensive and not readily available in most departments. Hence after the initial period of observation, the trainee is put to the test on the patient with the mentor standing by to take care of any issue before a mishap occurs. Mentioned below is one way of training the resident.

*Step 1*: In the initial 10-20 cases, allow the trainee to do the preliminary cystoscopy, assess the prostate and then pass the resectoscope with prior urethral dilatation or Otis urethrotomy depending on the caliber of the meatus.

*Step 2*: The mentor completes the resection and allows the trainee to clear the prostatic chips and achieve complete hemostasis and place the catheter.

*Step 3*: The trainee is allowed to resect the middle lobe. One of the problems to minimize is undermining the trigone. To prevent this sometimes it is useful to carry out two transurethral incisions of the prostate at 5 o'clock and 7 o'clock positions. The incision exposes the deeper limit of the resection on either side of the middle lobe. This is then used as the landmark to resect the middle lobe. Once confidence has been gained the above step can be omitted. At this time the resectoscope is positioned 1–2 cm distal to the bladder neck and base of the median lobe and resection is begun taking long smooth chips. Care must be taken to avoid cutting out large chunks of tissue as there is a risk of the lobe getting detached prematurely and floating into the bladder. In the early stage it is advisable to activate the current then begin to engage the tissue to enable resection. Multiple such excursions are need in a planned sequential manner to resect the median lobe.

*Step 4*: Resection of the median lobe and one lateral lobe. The lateral lobes can be resected using either of the techniques. In the Barnes technique the resection proceeds in a clockwise manner to the right lobe from 6 o'clock to 12 o'clock by taking loop excursions from the bladder neck region to the verumontanum either in single long sweeps if the prostate is small or in multiple smaller slivers if large. Hemostasis is achieved by the trainee and if things are proceeding to a plan and with no problems, he continues to resect the left lobe starting from the 6 o'clock and proceeding in an anticlockwise manner to the 12 o'clock position to meet the point of the earlier resection of the right lobe.

In the Nesbit technique (Figs. 8.8A to D) the resection is begun at 12 o'clock just inside the bladder neck exposing these fibers and working in the groove thus created in an anticlockwise manner detaching the entire right or left lobe from the bladder neck to the verumontanum. The lateral lobe once detached in this manner falls onto the floor of the prostatic urethra and one can then resect the fallen lobe up to and thus exposing the verumontanum. A similar technique is employed for the other side. The verumontanum is the distal limit of the resection.

*Resection near the apex*: There are some reports to indicate that leaving tissue at the prostatic apex helps in preventing retrograde ejaculation. Nevertheless most resectionists would aim to clean the region of the prostatic apex adequately. This is sometimes best achieved by lowering the height of the operating table, going up on the operating stool and looking down at the apex rather than looking at it tangentially. If an O'Connor drape (Fig. 8.11) has been placed prior to the resection, then finger in the rectum helps in elevating the prostate enabling adequate resection. The distal sphincter is always distal to the distal extent of the prostate even if it is going beyond the verumontanum.

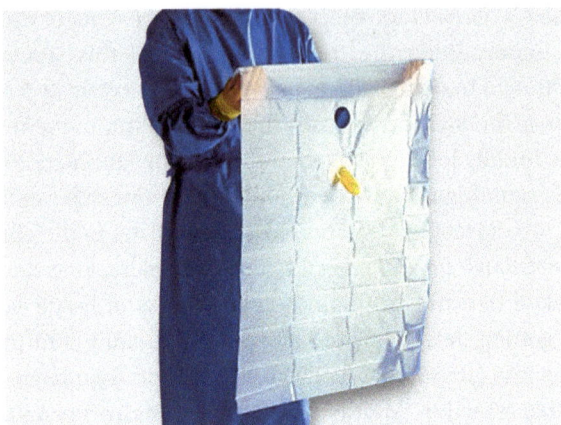

**Fig. 8.11:** O'connor drape.

*Step 5*: While it is necessary to carry out a near complete resection, in real terms, there are always some tags of tissue left over and it may be necessary to smoothen out the fossa to ensure good healing. It is a good idea to empty the bladder and have a look at the collapsed fossa to know if there is any residual tissue; overdistending the bladder will always give the impression that all prostate has been resected. Stopping the irrigation and examining the fossa will also help identify venous bleeders. Arterial bleeders are best coagulated at the time they are seen.

After one is satisfied that all prostate has been resected the chips from the bladder are evacuated, the integrity of the trigone and the ureteral orifices are ascertained and hemostasis is ensured. Hemostasis is ensured in a systematic manner starting from the bladder neck to the verumontanum. One area which is not infrequently missed is the anterior lobe at 2 o'clock and 11 o'clock positions.

The blood pressure is checked to ensure that it is stable prior to removing the resectoscope and inserting the catheter. If there has been an inadvertent undermining of the trigone there is a tendency for the catheter to not slide into the bladder. If this is the case then the catheter is placed either under vision over a guidewire or by using a Maryfield introducer. Most urologists insert a three-way Foley catheter and connect to continuous irrigation for 24 hours. If one is happy then a standard two-way catheter is used and the patient hydrated intravenously or by allowing oral fluids. Some urologists administer a dose of Frusemide or mannitol just prior to completing the resection to ensure a copious urine flow.

Make sure that when you send the patient to the postoperative ward that the urine is reasonably clear and patient hemodynamically stable so that you can get a good night's sleep.

# IRRIGATING SOLUTIONS DURING TRANSURETHRAL RESECTION OF THE PROSTATE

## Introduction

Endoscopic surgery in genitourinary tract requires the use of an irrigating fluid to gently dilate mucosal spaces and to remove blood and cut tissue from the operating field. There are several different irrigating fluids available commercially and it might be difficult to know which one to use. The choice tends to be governed largely by tradition, although the price and properties of the fluid also play a role. The pharmacological effects of the fluid become important whenever it is absorbed by the patient. The average rate of fluid absorption during TURP is 20 mL/minute. However, adverse reactions to irrigating fluids have not been documented as they have for drugs. Most irrigating fluids were developed when the documentation of safety was much less important than it is today.

## History

Sterile water was used as the irrigating fluid during the early years of TURP. However, obscure reactions with postoperative hemoglobinuria sometimes occurred and severe cases even led to death. In 1947, urologists realized that the absorption of the irrigating fluid into the circulation through severed prostatic veins must be the cause of the hemolysis. As electrolytes do not allow cutting by electrocautery, one or several nonelectrolyte solutes capable of preventing hemolysis were then added to the irrigating fluid.

Glycine was the first suggested as suitable; this amino acid is an endogenous substance, transparent in an iso-osmotic (2.2%) solution, and reasonably cheap. In 1948, Nesbit used 1.1% glycine in 230 consecutive cases and found no hemolysis. In his earlier resection, Nesbit used 10–25 L of distilled water for TURP. He realized that this caused significant problems including hemolysis. The other irrigating fluids used today, mannitol and mixtures of sorbitol and mannitol, were introduced somewhat later. The only further development in the composition of irrigating fluids since the early 1950s is the addition of ethanol up to a concentration of 1%, which allows fluid absorption to be monitored by expired-breath ethanol tests.

Despite their non-hemolytic properties, absorption of the new irrigating fluids continued to be associated with adverse events which were often summarized as "transurethral resection reactions" (TUR syndrome). The clinical descriptions of this syndrome from the mid-1950s are still the cornerstones of our view of the risks associated with the use of irrigating fluids.

## IDEAL IRRIGATION FLUID

An ideal irrigation fluid should be transparent, isotonic, nonconductive, nonhemolytic, nonmetabolized, nontoxic, inexpensive, and sterile. However, an ideal irrigation fluid is still unavailable. There are many irrigation fluids. Each has its own merits and demerits:

**Irrigation fluids:**
- Sterile water
- Glycine
- Mannitol
- Sorbitol
- Glucose
- Normal saline
- Ringer lactate.

Glycine and sterile water are the most widely used irrigating fluids in urological endoscopic surgeries.

## Sterile Water

Sterile water has many qualities of an ideal irrigating fluid. The disadvantage is its extreme hypotonicity, causing hemolysis, dilutional hyponatremia, shock, and renal failure.

## Glycine

Glycine is a nonessential amino acid that was introduced in 1948 as an irrigating fluid. It lacks allergic reactions and available at low cost. It is used in concentrations of 1.2%, 1.5% and 2.2%. Glycine is isotonic with plasma only at a concentration of 2.2%, but the side effects of glycine at this concentration are more. The osmolality of 1.5% glycine is 230 mOsm/L compared to serum osmolality of 290 mOsm/L and hence cardiovascular and renal toxicities can occur at this concentration also. Further lowering of the concentration of glycine can lead to more complications due to hypotonicity and hence cannot be used for irrigation purposes. The distinct advantage of 1.5% glycine over sterile water is its tendency to cause less hemolysis and renal failure. The plasma concentration is 0.3 mmol/L, which is raised 25-fold on administration of 1 L of this fluid. The half-life is dose-dependent, which is probably due to intracellular accumulation of glycine. Penetration into central nervous system is restricted, but may be clinically important. Elimination of glycine occurs primarily in the liver due to metabolism into ammonia. Around 5–10% of an excess dose is excreted unchanged in urine, promoting an osmotic diuresis. Visual disturbances correlate with plasma glycine concentration of 5–8 mmol/L, whereas higher concentrations produce transient blindness. Plasma concentrations above 20 mmol/L were associated with fatal TUR syndromes.

## Mannitol

Mannitol is an isomer of glucose. It is used at concentration of 3% and 5%. Though does not have the toxicities of glycine, drives water out of cells and may enhance circulatory overloading. The cost of mannitol is also higher compared to glycine. The elimination of mannitol through kidney will be decreased in patients with impaired renal function.

## Sorbitol

Another irrigant used in TURP. It is metabolized to fructose and glucose in the liver and has a distribution half-life of 6 minutes and a terminal half-life of 33 minutes. Like glycine, 5–10% is excreted unchanged in the urine. The visibility is poor with its use and hence it is not used widely.

### Cytal

Cytal, a mixture of sorbitol 2.7% and mannitol 0.54% widely used in USA as an irrigating fluid, has not gained popularity in India due to its high cost and nonavailability.

## Glucose

This is not a widely used irrigating fluid since glucose produces tissue charring at the site of resection and associated hyperglycemia produced when glucose is absorbed into the circulation. It also causes stickiness of surgeon's gloves and instruments. When it is used, it is used at concentration between 2.5–4%.

### Urea

It is used at a concentration of 1%. This produces urea crystallization on the instruments during resection and hence not preferred.

## Normal Saline

Normal saline is used for irrigation with the advent of bipolar resection. It is the only iso-osmolar irrigant used. Although cerebral edema is unlikely, infusion of volumes more than 25 mL/kg for more than 15 minutes might result in mental changes and swellings. Moreover, it can cause hyperchloremic acidosis. It results in more plasma volume expansion, thereby pulmonary edema can be a sequelae.

# REFERENCES

1. Orandi A. Transurethral Incision of Prostate (TUIP): 646 cases in 15 Years—a Chronological Appraisal. Br J Urol. 1985;57:703-7.
2. Mobb GE, Moisey CU. Long-term follow-up of unilateral bladder neck incision. Br J Urol. 1988;62:160-2.
3. Turner-Warwick R, Whiteside CG, Worth PH, et al. A urodynamic view of the clinical problems associated with bladder neck dysfunction and its treatment by endoscopic incision and trans-trigonal posterior prostatectomy. Br J Urol. 1973;45:44-59.
4. Mebust WK, Holtgrewe HL, Cockett AT, et al. Transurethral prostatectomy: immediate and postoperative complications. A cooperative study of 13 participating institutions evaluating 3,885 patients. J Urol. 1989;141:243-7.
5. Agrawal MS, Aron M, Goel R. Hemiresection of the prostate: short-term randomized comparison with standard transurethral resection. J Endourol. 2005;19:868-72.
6. McGowan SW, Smith GF. Anaesthesia for transurethral prostatectomy. A comparison of spinal intradural analgesia with two methods of general anaesthesia. Anaesthesia. 1980;35:847-53.
7. Nielsen KK, Andersen K, Asbjørn J, et al. Blood loss in transurethral prostatectomy: epidural versus general anaesthesia. Int Urol Nephrol. 1987;19:287-92.
8. Kulb TB, Kamer M, Lingeman JE, et al. Prevention of post-prostatectomy vesical neck contracture by prophylactic vesical neck incision. J Urol. 1987;137:230-1.

# Chapter 9

# Transurethral Enucleation and Resection of Prostate

*Mallikarjuna Chiruvella, Md Taif Bendigeri*

## INTRODUCTION

The management of benign prostatic hyperplasia (BPH) has seen a significant shift in the approach from the days of open prostatectomy to the present day. The surgical principle of treatment in the era of open prostatectomy had been enucleation of the adenoma from the peripheral zone of prostate utilizing the plane between the surgical capsule/pseudocapsule and the adenoma. After the advent of endoscopic era, the principle to achieve similar clearance of adenoma was applied in various manners. The most important is transurethral resection of the prostate (TURP), which has been regarded as gold standard of endoscopic treatment of BPH for several decades. The replication of the principle of enucleation through endoscopic approach has been the much awaited improvement over TURP. This provides twin advantages of following the best possible surgical treatment principle for BPH and maintaining the improved outcomes in regards of postoperative morbidity of endoscopic treatment modality. Hence we can safely infer that endoscopic enucleation is the rightful gold standard for surgical treatment of BPH.

Endoscopic enucleation can be achieved by using lasers such as holmium and thulium or bipolar energy. Irrespective of the energy which is being utilized, the most important criteria remains achievement of enucleation endoscopically. The entire spectrum of endoscopic enucleation has nevertheless been made more popular and exciting by the holmium laser. The major hurdle which stood in the path of universal applicability of these new lasers was the astronomical initial cost of investment and maintenance, especially from the perspective of developing nations. This led to the improvization of the regular bipolar instrument set to achieve the goal of endoscopic enucleation without any additional new cost. This procedure is known by various nomenclature such as transurethral enucleation of prostate with bipolar (TUEB), plasmakinetic enucleation, transurethral enucleation-resection of prostate, bipolar enucleation of prostate and so on.

The procedure of transurethral enucleation and resection of prostate (TUERP) has been the next major improvization in this journey of endoscopic enucleation. This attains significance mainly due to the fact that it does away with the need for a morcellator which is essential with conventional complete enucleation. Hence, it further reduces the cost involved in achieving the goal of endoscopic enucleation.

In this chapter, we will be highlighting the various aspects of this procedure, starting from the instruments required, various methods of performing this procedure, results, and complications, limitations, and road ahead.

## INSTRUMENTS

The instruments required for performing transurethral enucleation of prostate using bipolar energy is very similar to that used for the bipolar TURP procedure. The Figure 9.1 shows the usual arrangement of instruments needed for the procedure.

There are a few important aspects to be noted in the instruments used for this procedure:
- The major change in the instruments for this procedure as compared to that used for a regular bipolar TURP is the specially designed loop. The procedure can be performed using the regular loops as well, however the modifications in the loop design make the enucleation procedure easier to learn and replicate. The loops combine a mechanical component along with the conventional active component. The mechanical part is inactive and steadier. It makes the step of mechanical separation of the adenoma from the pseudocapsule easier by allowing the surgeon to visualize the exact site of separation of adenoma directly. If the enucleation is to be

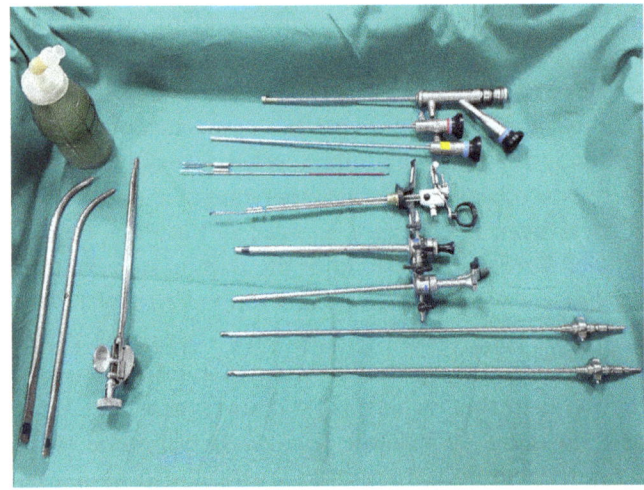

**Fig. 9.1:** Arrangement of the instruments required for bipolar enucleation.

performed using conventional loops, then the separation of adenoma has to be achieved mainly by the beak of the sheath and hence the exact site of separation is not in full vision and the surgeon has to rely on his three-dimensional orientation and haptic feel of the process as well. However, a beginner will need some time to shift the point of focus, from the active loop during TURP to the inactive loop during enucleation (Fig. 9.2).

Different manufactures achieve this target of combining the active element of loop and a steady mechanical inactive element for enucleation through various designs (Figs. 9.3 and 9.4).

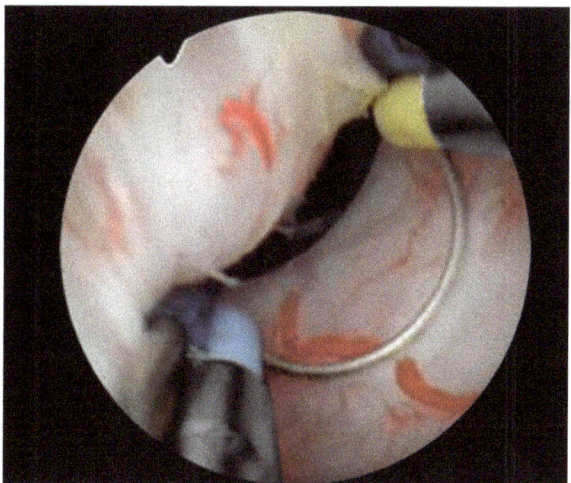

**Fig. 9.2:** Endoscopic image showing the advantage of using modified loops for transurethral enucleation of prostate with bipolar (TUEB) which enable to see the exact site of enucleation.

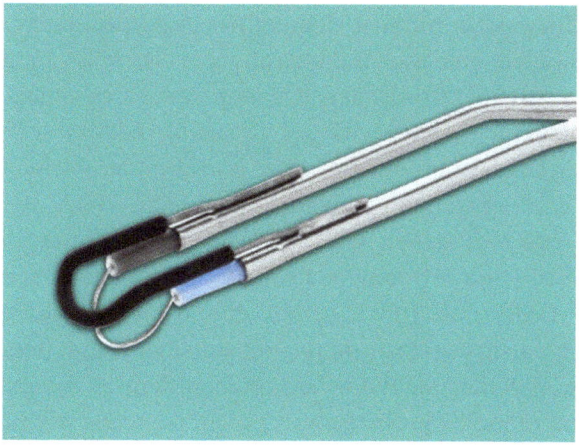

**Fig. 9.3:** Transurethral enucleation of prostate with bipolar (TUEB) loop from Olympus.

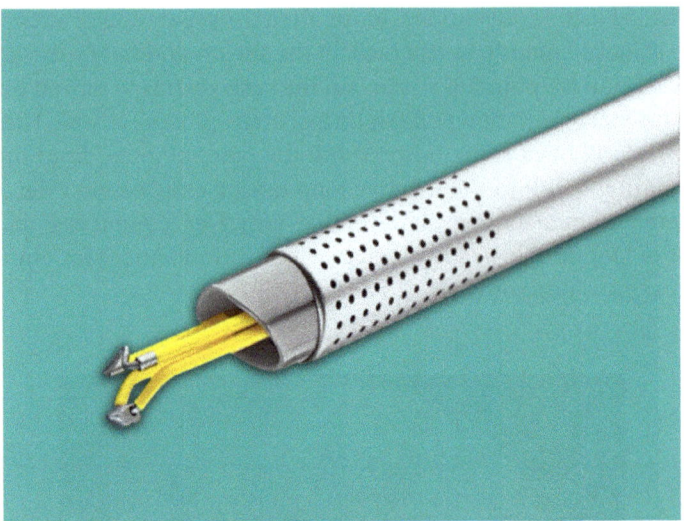

**Fig. 9.4:** Loop from Karl Storz for bipolar enucleation of prostate.

Irrespective of the design type of loop used, the target and the principle remain the same. Some surgeons have extended the use of mushroom/button electrode as well for the same purpose (Fig. 9.5).

Another important aspect of the loop design is the longer length as compared to the normal loop. This makes the mechanical component and the active component to protrude out of the sheath even in resting position of a passive working element resectoscope set or maximal withdrawn position of an active working element resectoscope set (Figs. 9.6 and 9.7).

The main advantage of having a longer loop is that the surgeon can change his grip of holding the instrument assembly and have his fingers free especially with passive working element resectoscope. This is essential for an ergonomically better way of enucleation. It also helps in automatically changing the point of focus from active loop to the mechanical loop. It also helps in avoiding the tendency to use a pushing movement on loop using fingers during enucleation. The main aim is to keep the assembly still during the maneuver of separation of adenoma (Figs. 9.8 and 9.9).

- The telescope most widely used for TURP is 30°. However, while using the modified loops for doing enucleation using bipolar energy, we will need a 12° telescope. This is mainly due to the fact that the modified loops have the mechanical component at a higher level (lesser degree of angulation with the longitudinal axis of loop stem) as compared to active component of the loop. Hence, using a 30° telescope will not have both the components of the loop within the field of vision.

# Transurethral Enucleation and Resection of Prostate

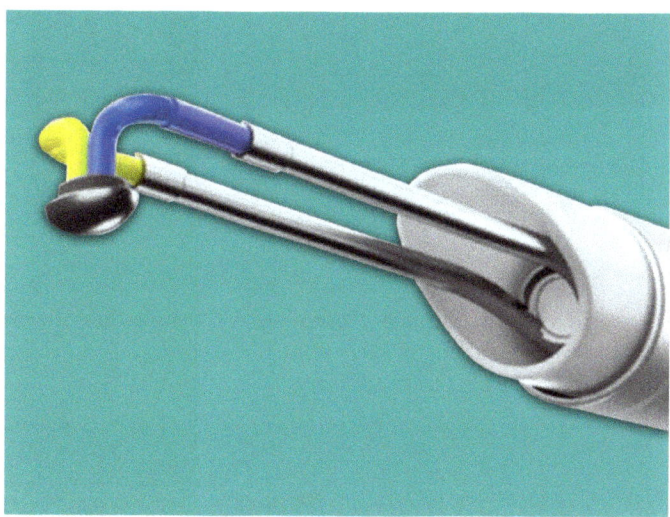

**Fig. 9.5:** Mushroom button electrode from Olympus.

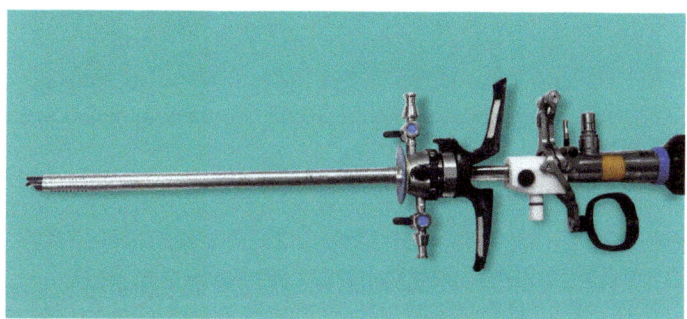

**Fig. 9.6:** Transurethral enucleation of prostate with bipolar (TUEB) loop in passive element resting position.

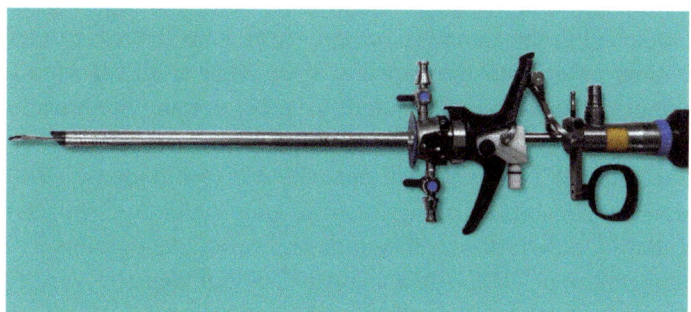

**Fig. 9.7:** Transurethral enucleation of prostate with bipolar (TUEB) loop in active working element resting position.

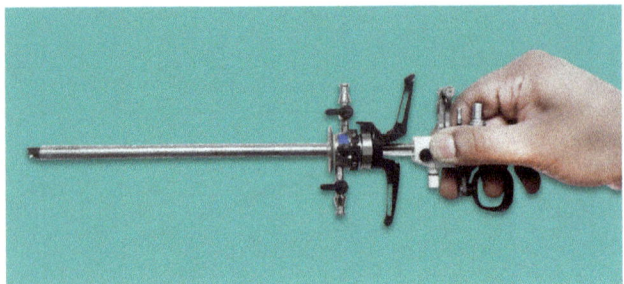

**Fig. 9.8:** Modified grip of instrument assembly for transurethral enucleation of prostate with bipolar (TUEB).

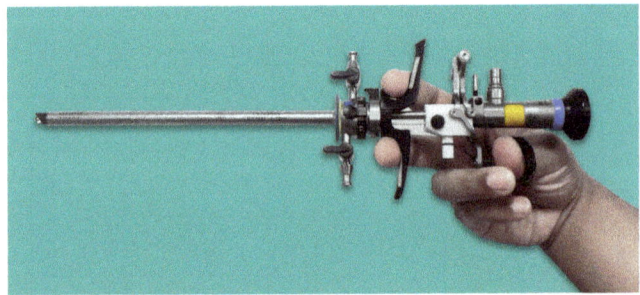

**Fig. 9.9:** Conventional grip of instrument assembly for transurethral resection of the prostate (TURP).

## TECHNIQUE OF PERFORMING TRANSURETHRAL ENUCLEATION OF PROSTATE WITH BIPOLAR

Transurethral enucleation of prostate with bipolar was advocated and popularized by Liu C et al. to achieve outcomes similar to laser enucleation. The technique of enucleation was performed using the standard resection sheath and was called "TUERP" by them. Subsequently, Nakagawa modified the procedure by introducing the "TUEB loop" which had a specially designed spatula attached to the standard Tungsten wire loop electrode to enucleate the adenoma away from the capsule. Since Neill et al. reported the first bipolar enucleation of prostate, there have been many modifications, but no standardized technique is available, that can be adopted and emulated like the traditional TURP. We will describe our technique of TUEB which is safe and easy to start learning the art of enucleation and simultaneously also highlight the various modifications and variations possible in TUEB.

The procedure of TUEB mainly consists of four steps:
1. Defining the anatomical landmarks for enucleation
2. Making grooves in floor and roof
3. Enucleation of adenoma
4. Morcellation/resection.

## Step 1: Defining the Anatomical Landmarks for Enucleation

The initial step begins with a thorough urethrocystoscopy as done at the beginning for any endoscopic procedure for prostate. The enlargement pattern of the adenoma is assessed. The technique differs slightly if there is trilobar enlargement pattern of the adenoma as compared to bilobar pattern. The prostatic length is assessed. It is essential to develop a baseline three-dimensional impression of the gland at the start of the procedure, so that the extent of enucleation maneuvers required can be anticipated. The relation of the distal extent of the adenoma is relation to the external sphincter is assessed. The white line of Hilton which is formed at the junction of the adenoma and mucosa is more relevant landmark as compared to verumontanum, especially in larger glands wherein the adenoma extends distally beyond the verumontanum. The adenoma mucosa junction is marked all around with electrocautery to form the distal limit of enucleation (Figs. 9.10 to 9.15).

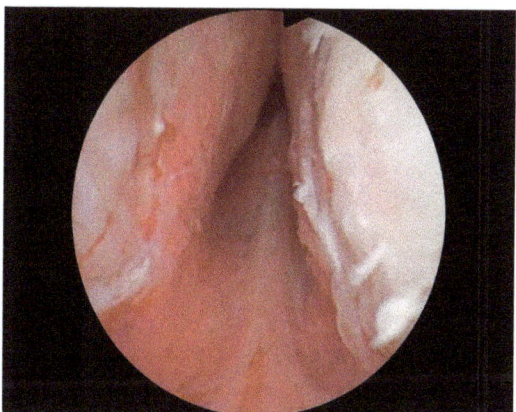

**Fig. 9.10:** Assessment of the gland and identification of distal extent of adenoma mucosa junction.

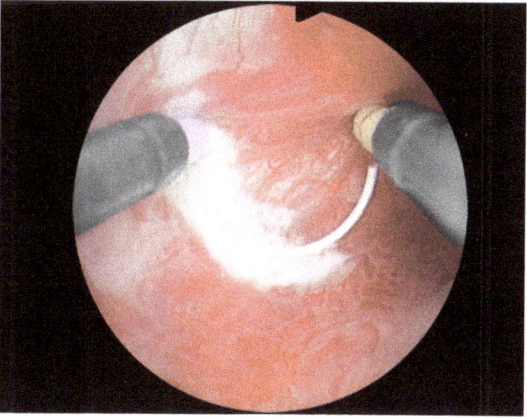

**Fig. 9.11:** Mucosal marking on right lobe at adenoma mucosa junction.

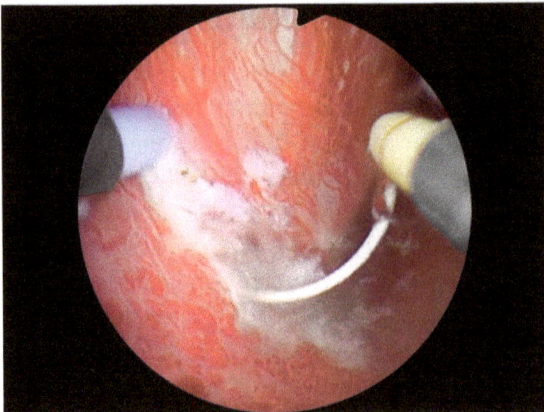

**Fig. 9.12:** Deepening of the mucosal marking with short bursts of energy to incise the mucosa.

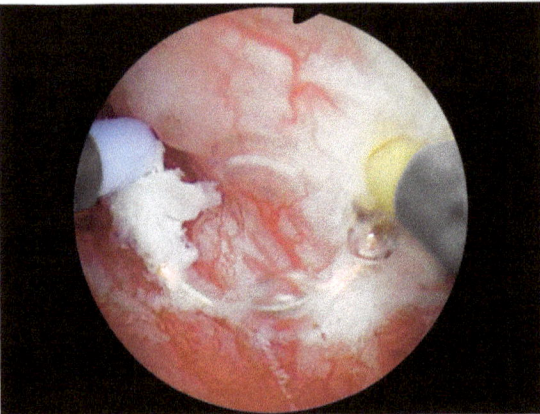

**Fig. 9.13:** Mucosal marking on left lobe at adenoma mucosa junction.

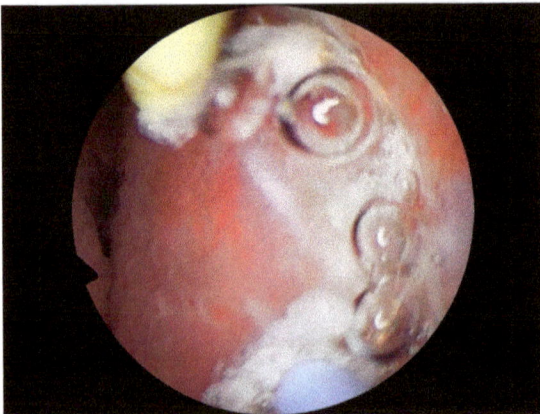

**Fig. 9.14:** Completing the mucosal marking all around to define the distal extent of the procedure.

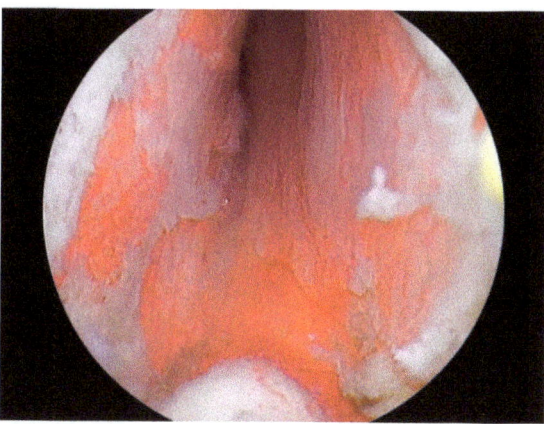

**Fig. 9.15:** Distal circumferential mucosal marking defining the distal limit of enucleation.

## Step 2: Making Grooves in Floor and Roof (Figs. 9.16 and 9.17)

Next step involves making grooves in the floor and roof. The groove in the floor can be done at 5 o'clock or 7 o'clock for bilobar enlargement. In case of trilobar enlargement with a large median lobe, there are two options. It can be done either in a way similar to bilobar gland using single groove and clubbing of the median lobe with one lateral gland or the other option is to deal with the median lobe separately from the lateral lobes which will require both 5 o'clock and 7 o'clock grooves to be made. If median lobe is separated from both lateral lobes then median lobe will need to be enucleated separately. In case of moderately enlarged median lobes, it can be resected off in between the two grooves and rest of enucleation carried out as bilobar gland.

This is followed by making groove in the roof at 12 o'clock position. The grooves extend from the bladder neck to the distal mucosal marking in length. The depth of resection of the groove stops well short of the capsule. The grooves are beneficial in several ways:

- The grooves act as essential landmarks during the process of enucleation by helping in maintaining the orientation of the exact position of progress with regards to the adenoma. This becomes helpful especially in very large glands; while working in the plane of enucleation there will be no other immediate landmarks available to gauge the exact site and progress of enucleation prior to reaching the bladder neck.
- The grooves separate the lateral lobes from each other so that they can be enucleated independently and pushed back easily into the bladder across the bladder neck if morcellation is intended. This is especially of

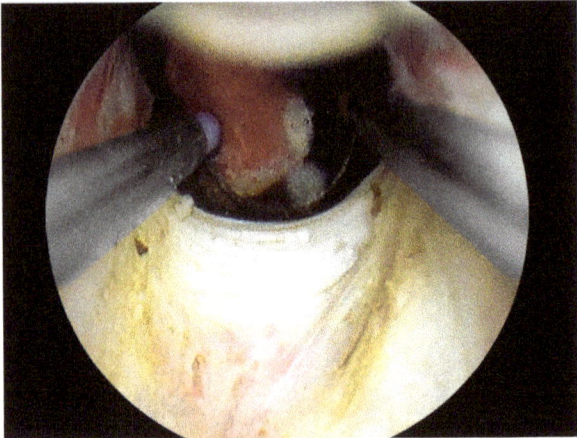

**Fig. 9.16:** Groove in the floor of the prostate.

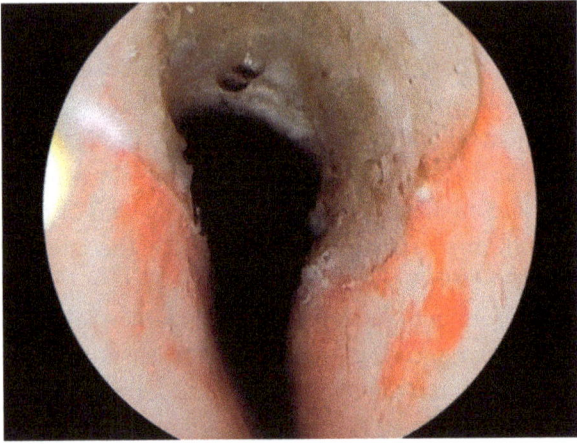

**Fig. 9.17:** Groove on roof.

significance when the gland is very large to be pushed intact across the bladder neck.
- The grooves help in improving the flow of irrigant fluid and hence achieving improvement in the vision.

## Step 3: Enucleation of Adenoma (Figs. 9.18 to 9.25)

The process of enucleating the adenoma begins at the distal mucosal marking made initially. The mucosa is incised with short bursts of cutting electrocautery all around. Once the mucosa is incised the plane between

# Transurethral Enucleation and Resection of Prostate

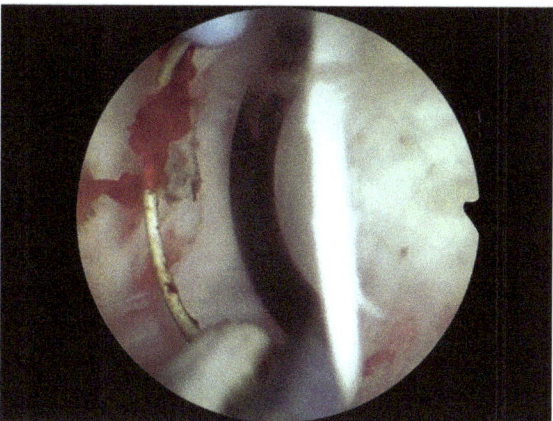

**Fig. 9.18:** Enucleation of right lobe at about 8 o'clock position.

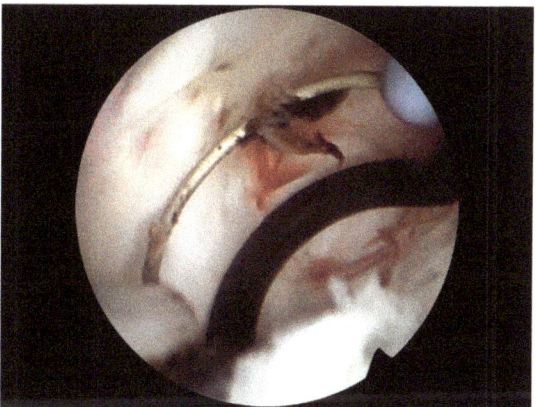

**Fig. 9.19:** Progress of enucleation of right lobe at about 11 o'clock position.

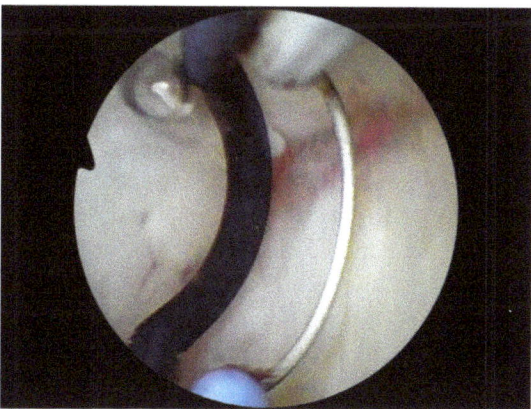

**Fig. 9.20:** Enucleation of left lobe at 5 o'clock position.

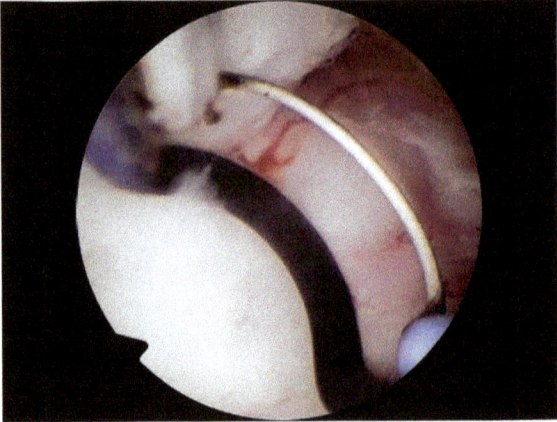

**Fig. 9.21:** Enucleation of left lobe at 2 o'clock position.

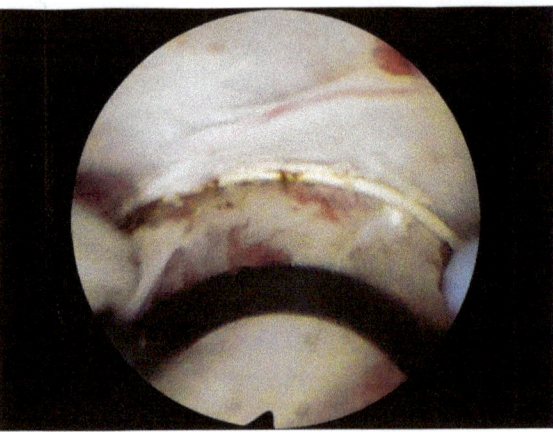

**Fig. 9.22:** Enucleation plane proceeding toward the bladder neck at 12 o'clock position.

the adenoma and the compressed peripheral gland is identified with gentle manual stretch over the adenoma. The enucleation is carried forward in the plane between surgical capsule and the adenoma. It proceeds anteriorly to circumferentially delineate the plane at the distal extent and then start proceeding proximally toward the bladder neck at the roof. The enucleation requires separation of the adenoma using the mechanical component of the loop and any bleeder encountered is controlled with the active component of loop. It is easier to try and reach the bladder neck at roof (12 o'clock) since the distance of prostate is shortest at that level and with least amount of gland. The bladder neck is identified by the appearance of transparent mucosa immediately prior to entering the bladder. The bladder mucosa

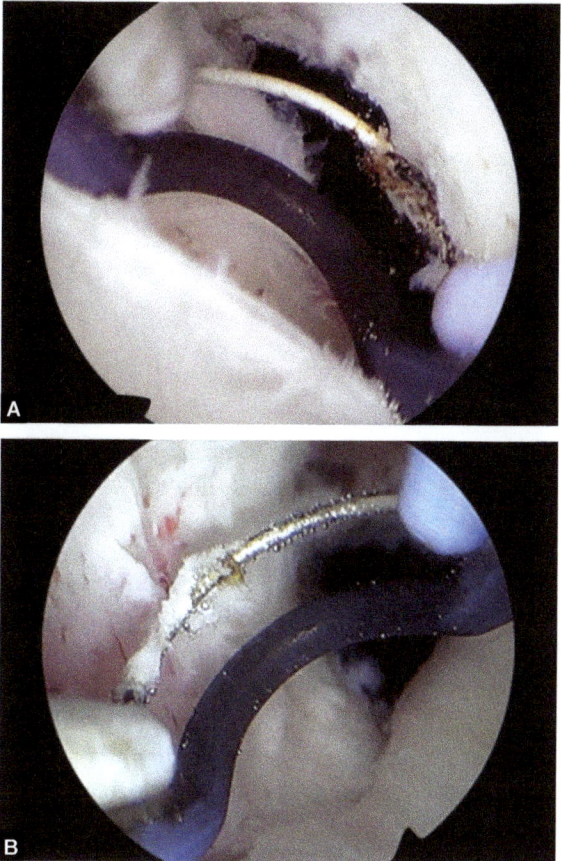

**Figs. 9.23A and B:** Separation of adenoma from the bladder at level of bladder neck circumferentially.

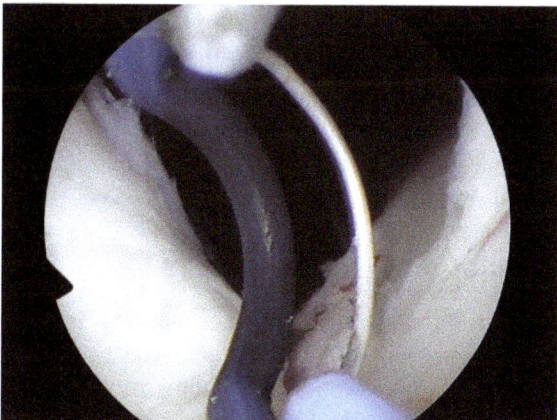

**Fig. 9.24:** Adenoma almost completely separated from the capsule at the proximal level of bladder neck.

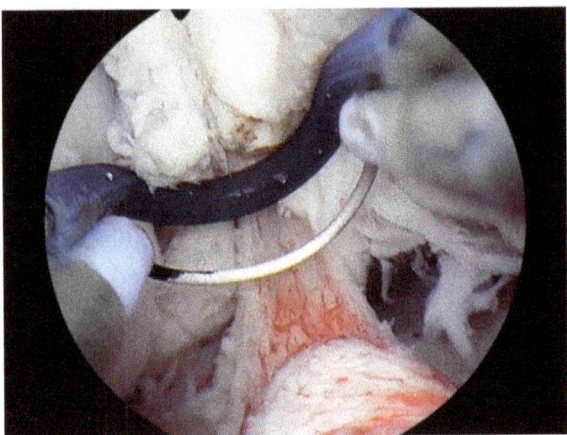

**Fig. 9.25:** At the end of enucleation, the avascular enucleated adenoma remains attached only by a small segment of tissue at verumontanum.

is incised and the plane of enucleation communicates with the bladder lumen. This marks completion of enucleation plane at this segment of gland. Another important clue to assess the proximity of bladder neck during enucleation is the appearance of major feeding vessels to the adenoma which enter the adenoma near bladder neck. It is this control of vessels at the entry point that makes the adenoma avascular. Once the plane of separation is completed with entry into bladder at the level of roof, the enucleation plane is carried down circumferentially at the level of bladder neck all around, from the roof down to the floor, to take the plane of enucleation past the 6 o'clock groove. This process is similarly repeated moving more distally and separating the adenoma at each level from roof to the floor. As the enucleation proceeds from bladder neck distally, the adenoma is finally separated over entire its length and remains attached only with a short attachment of gland near the verumontanum. The process is repeated similarly on the other lobe. Once the enucleation is completed, the two lobes will be avascular, and separated from the surgical capsule all around, with only a small attachment near verumontanum holding them in place for in situ resection.

## Step 4: Morcellation/Resection

Once the process of enucleation is over, we will be left with an avascular gland which needs retrieval. This can be achieved by either morcellation or in situ resection. Conventional enucleation procedures have utilized complete enucleation of the gland and pushing it off into the bladder and then performing the morcellation. The most important point to be kept in mind before morcellation is begun is to have completely controlled hemostasis and a clear unhindered vision. Any impairment of vision due to bleeding increases the risk of bladder perforation significantly. Morcellation needs the separate set of instruments for this step and its associated issues. Hence, in situ resection of the enucleated avascular adenoma while keeping it attached at a small section is preferred. It obviates the need for the morcellator setup. While resecting the enucleated adenoma, few points have to be kept in mind (Fig. 9.26):

- The resection can proceed from lumen toward the enucleated plane or vice versa starting from the enucleated plane and proceeding toward the urethral lumen. The second technique is easier and faster. So negotiating the instrument in the enucleation plane right up to the bladder neck and proceeding with resection from periphery towards center is preferred.
- Toward the end of the resection, there is usually a nagging issue of residual flaps of tissue which needs to be trimmed. This arises due to an onion peeling effect during the process of enucleation and finding the proper plane. These flaps have to carefully leveled to the surface. This is extremely important because of the possibility of a bleeder underneath the flap which can open up in postoperative period.
- At the distal end of resection, there may be a mucosal flap which gets lifted off at the roof. Care has to be taken not to be overenthusiastic in resecting this flap due to the proximity to sphincter and the innocuous nature of the mucosal flap.
- There may be few residual nodules of the adenoma which can be left behind during enucleation especially near the apex. Care has to be taken to resect these nodules else these may cause impaired results and recurrence of obstruction at apex.

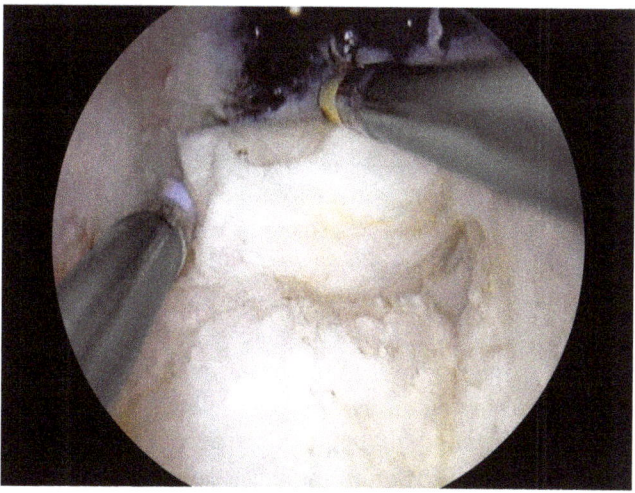

**Fig. 9.26:** Resection of the avascular enucleated adenoma.

## VARIATIONS IN TECHNIQUES

There are numerous variations in the technique to achieve the enucleation:
- Enucleation can be done without the use of any modified loops as was initially described and popularized by Liu et al. The beak of the sheath acts as the enucleating part.
- Enucleation has been described with usage of monopolar energy as well. However, most of the recent techniques use bipolar energy.
- Enucleation with in situ resection can be done with keeping the adenoma attached even at the bladder neck for a short segment. Care has to be taken not to keep the segment of attachment too small else there will be wobbling of the adenoma making resection a tough task. There have been variations of keeping the attachment at the distal part of the adenoma on lateral aspect and enucleating the rest of adenoma.
- Enucleation and resection can also be done in a pattern of completing enucleation and resection of one lobe completely and then proceeding to enucleation of other side. It provides few additional benefits. The space for maneuvering increases significantly after the resection and clearance one lobe from the fossa. In case of any major inadvertent event during the early part of surgery, the procedure can be terminated early as compared to having proceeded with enucleation of both lobes simultaneously.
- There have reports of using mushroom button electrode as well for achieving the enucleation.
- Several different patterns of modifications of loops add to the variety in ways of achieving enucleation.
- There is an ejaculation preserving TUEB also hypothesized which attributes reduced incidence of retrograde ejaculation to preserving a small strip of tissue adjacent to verumontanum and indirectly preserving a small muscle encircling the verumontanum which is needed for antegrade ejaculation.

## COMPLICATIONS

Most of the complications of TUEB are similar to those encountered during TURP. During enucleation, the most common complication encountered is capsular perforation. According to Maurmayer, capsular perforation can be graded accordingly as: (1) threatened perforation; (2) covered perforation; (3) free perforation; and (4) subtrigonal perforation. Irrespective of the technique of enucleation, capsular perforations are encountered during the initial learning phase when the amount of pressure needed and the three-dimensional orientations is not yet well-coordinated and in small prostate glands where the glands are more fibrous and firmly adherent. The conventional wisdom of more difficulty to enucleate small glands in open prostatectomy holds true for endoscopic enucleation as well. Capsular perforations of higher grade like free and subtrigonal perforation may require prolonged urethral catheterization. The incidence of perforation may range from 2% to 15% in various series.

Hematuria and blood loss have been shown to be significantly less in TUEB as compared to TURP. In TUEB, the specially designed electrode enables to achieve excellent coagulation of the bleeders during the process of enucleation. Because of the early control of bleeding, visibility remains excellent throughout the procedure. Hemoglobin drop of 0.3-1.2 g% has been reported in literature.

Incontinence of urine following enucleation has been reported with holmium laser enucleation of the prostate (HoLEP) and TUEB. Early transient incontinence rate following TUEB in reported literature is 2-10%; which is less than HoLEP (4-36%). However, persistent stress incontinence following both TUEB and HoLEP is rare (0-4.5%). Generally following TUR, early incontinence of urine is attributed to irritative symptoms due to resected prostatic fossa, detrusor instability or weakness and stretching of the external sphincter due to the enlarged prostate. Enucleation of a large adenoma extending close to the external sphincter may cause pronounced transient incontinence due to shearing trauma especially at the roof in 12 o'clock region. The incontinence usually resolves over a period of 1-6 months with conservative management like perineal exercises or anticholinergic medications. Other options include submucosal injection of dextranomer and hyaluronic acid at the level of external sphincter to improve the mucosal coaptation due to the bulking effect. Due diligence taken during marking the initial mucosal incision just proximal to the sphincter, by retaining adequate mucosa to avoid stretching or shearing injury to the external sphincter especially at 12 o'clock region, helps in reducing the rates of incontinence of urine.

The other complications inherent to endoscopic management of prostate such as postoperative stricture urethra, UTI, bladder neck contracture and retrograde ejaculation persist with TUEB as well. Retrograde ejaculation rates are being claimed to be reduced with ejaculation preserving modifications. Recurrence of bladder outlet obstruction post.

## CONCLUSION

Transurethral enucleation of prostate with bipolar allows enucleation of large adenomas in a single sitting, mimicking the conventional open enucleation of prostate while having all the advantages of a minimally invasive surgery. TUEB has less blood loss with minimal transfusion rates, fewer complications, shorter convalescence, acceptable continence rates and significant improvements in International Prostate Symptom Score (IPSS) and Qmax. However, there is a need for a long-term follow-up and a need for comparative studies with TURP and HoLEP to clarify the role of TUEB in the entire spectrum of endoscopic management of prostate.

# TRANSURETHRAL VAPORIZATION OF PROSTATE

## CONCEPT OF VAPORIZATION

The gold standard for minimally invasive treatment of prostate has been TURP for decades. However, TURP has been accompanied with its own share or complications though significantly less compared to the morbidities of open surgical procedures prior to it. One of the most dreaded complication of TURP has been bleeding. Several attempts were hence made to improvise upon the technique and instrumentation of TURP to reduce the bleeding and its morbidities. One of these attempts has been the development of vaporization of prostate. Several modifications have been introduced in the vaporization of prostate over past two decades since it was first used. It has been addressed by various abbreviations such as transurethral vaporization of prostate (TUVP), TVP, TUEVP, EVAP, PKVP, etc. The central idea remains the same and tries to achieve vaporization, desiccation and coagulation of prostate tissue.

Transurethral vaporization of prostate (TUVP) was first described by Kaplan and Te (1995). It combines the concepts of vaporization and desiccation. Desiccation is the drawing out of water from tissue and vaporization leads to evaporation of water from the cells. These work of different patterns or temperature and electrical energy settings.

## PRINCIPLE OF ACTION

The vaporization of prostate can be divided into two types: (1) electro-vaporization and (2) plasmakinetic vaporization. Electrovaporization utilized higher energy settings to achieve vaporization, desiccation, and coagulation. Plasmakinetic vaporization is based on the usage of plasma energy to achieve vaporization and coagulation.

With TUVP, two electrosurgical effects are combined: (1) vaporization and (2) desiccation. Vaporization steams tissue away using high heat and coagulation uses lower heat to dry out tissue. Other factors that matter are voltage production by the generator, the current density of the surface area of contact of the electrode, and the electrical resistance of the tissue being treated (Kaplan et al. 1998). The leading edge of the electrode is the point at which maximal efficiency for vaporization occurs and current density delivery. At the trailing edge of the electrode, there is a decrease in the delivery of current, lowering the power, and permitting tissue desiccation to occur. Therefore, vaporization occurs at the leading edge and desiccation occurs at the trailing edge (Kaplan et al. 1998).

Vaporization and desiccation depend on the hydration of the tissues, well hydrated ones vaporize and the drier ones desiccate. The electrical resistance also varies accordingly with drier tissues having higher resistance which needs higher power to overcome. Modern generators specifically designed for TUVP change the power delivered based on the tissue resistance. For TUVP, as compared to TURP, the cutting current power should be set to a maximum of 75% higher power. A minimal power delivery of 150 W is required for TUVP (van Swol et al. 1999).

## Electrode Design

The electrode design is very essential in achieving the vaporization effect. The features which are utilized to achieve better vaporization are:
- Larger surface area
- Ability to roll the electrode slowly
- Multiple grooves for increase in number of leading edges
- Variable thickness of loop, thin area for vaporization and thick one for desiccation.

These variations have been utilized by various companies with usage if different nomenclature (Figs. 9.27A and B).
- *Rollerball*: One of the initial electrodes for electrovaporization, useful however only for smaller glands due to its uniform surface.
- *Grooved rollerbar*: It consists of a bar that is 3 mm wide and 3 mm in diameter, which is composed of nickel-silver and insulated with Teflon (Vapor Trode, Circon-ACMI, Stamford, CT). It has more number of leading edges at which electrovaporization takes place, and this allows increased efficiency of vaporization to a wide contact area and thus to a larger volume of tissue (Narayan et al. 1996).

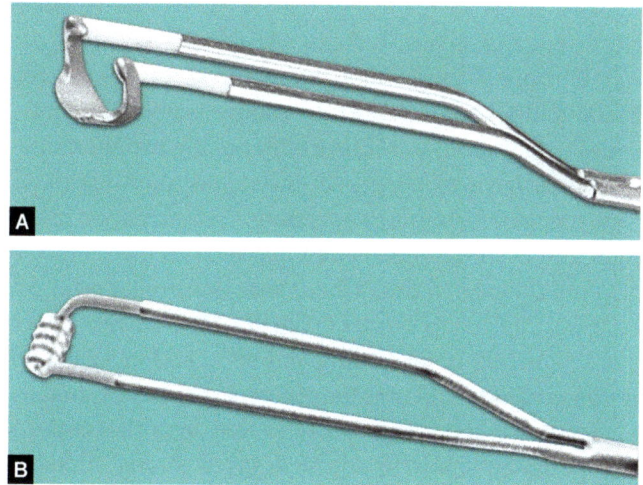

**Figs. 9.27A and B:** (A) Vaporcut electrode; and (B) Roller electrode.

- Wing EVAP (Richard Wolf, Germany) is a semicircular gold-plated wide loop that is wider and thicker than the standard TURP loop (Cabelin et al. 2000).
- *Vapor Tome (Circon-ACMI, Stamford, CT)*: A thick loop with grooves, giving a thin leading edge for vaporization and a thick trailing edge for desiccation.
- *The Wedge (Microvasive, Natick, MA)*: A smooth loop with the variable thickness principle for vaporization and desiccation.

Bipolar electrovaporization technology is the latest technology that has entered the electrovaporization arena. It works on plasmakinetic mechanism for vaporization and often referred to as plasmakinetic vaporization. It brings into picture all the advantages of plasma energy usage over conventional electrical energy. The loop design uses maximal surface area for large contact. Here the concept of leading edges does not exist. The surface of the loop rather does not come in complete contact with the tissues and it is the plasma generated at the surface that vaporizes the tissues. The various electrodes for plasma vaporization are:
- *Button electrode*: Provided by Gyrus/Olympus, it has large surface area with a mushroom-shaped built. It generates wide area of plasma and hence relatively faster compared to any previous vaporization electrodes. It does not have the limitation of slow and prolonged contact for vaporization and hence can be used for larger glands as well. It has been used for vaporization, vaporesection, and vapoenucleation uses (Figs. 9.28A and B).
- *ACMI hemielectrode*: It essentially similar to button electrode and works on similar principles (Fig. 9.29).

## TECHNIQUE

There have been two main techniques of utilizing the principle of vaporization. First one is pure vaporization and second one is combination of vaporization and resection known as vaporesection. The loop pattern of electrodes has been utilized to achieve either of the two methods. However, the roller patterns have relied purely on vaporization alone. The button electrodes are being used for pure vaporization, combination of vaporization and resection and even for enucleation as well.

*Vaporization*: The main point of focus here is the roller electrode element that is used instead of a loop element. The electrical current generator is set between 120 W and 300 W for cutting and 60 W and 75 W for coagulation. The settings however are different for different makes. A systematic process is followed and the roller electrode is moved over the entire surface of prostate to vaporize it. It should not be dragged through tissue and rather just rolled over the prostatic tissue with moderate pressure. Since the slow

# Transurethral Enucleation and Resection of Prostate

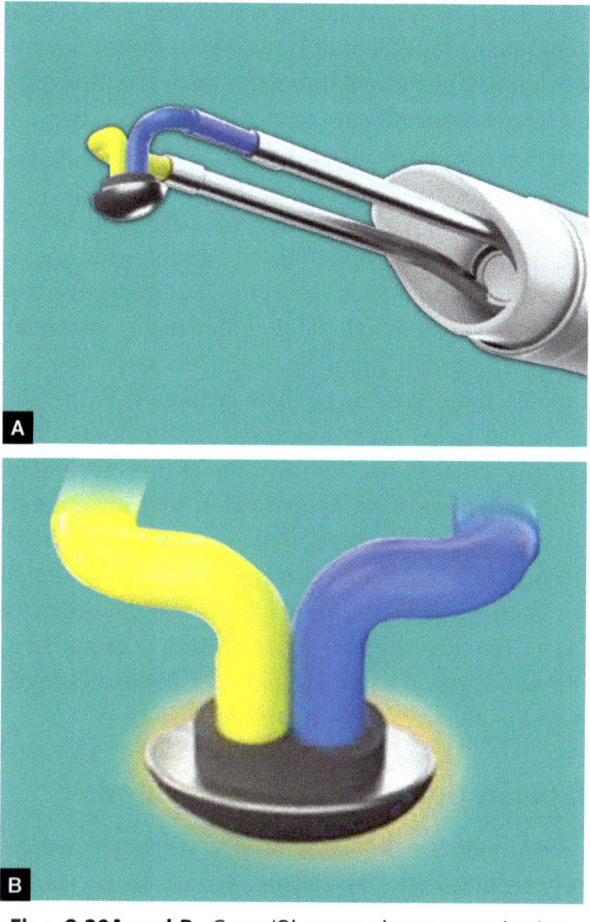

**Figs. 9.28A and B:** Gyrus/Olympus plasma vaporization.

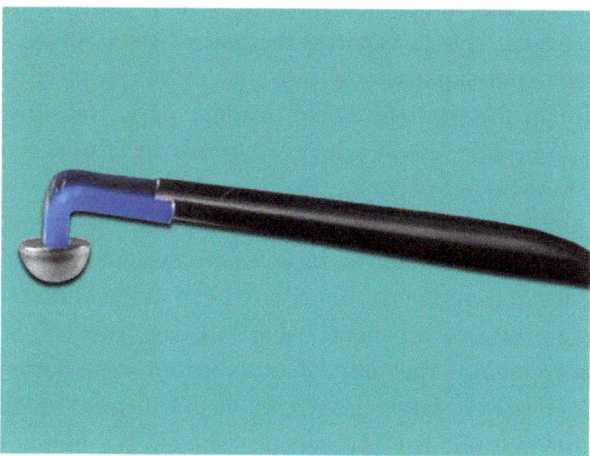

**Fig. 9.29:** ACMI hemielectrode.

motion of roller electrode is the basis for vaporization, the pace of procedure is slower as compared to resection. However, it should not be too slow or else a zone of char will be formed on surface of tissues making vaporization difficult. Because the tissue is being vaporized, there will be no specimen for pathology. If tissue is needed for evaluation, a standard loop can be used later.

*Vaporesection*: This is a combination of TURP and vaporization. The electrodes are the modified loops utilizing variables thickness and shapes for achieving vaporization and desiccation. The procedure is planned and carried out like a conventional TURP following a systematic sequence of resection. The important point that one has to remember is that the movements of the loop have to be slow swipes. It is the slower motion of the electrode that helps achieve optimal vaporization, desiccation, and coagulation of prostatic tissue. The slowing of the movements invariably slows down the resection pace as compared to conventional TURP and ends up with longer operative time. However, some time may be saved as a result of having clearer visualization if a deliberate systematic course of vaporesection is taken. Here the principle to be followed is "slow is clear and clear is fast". The advantage of vaporesection over pure vaporization is that it is faster and there is tissue available for histopathology. There is no need to change the electrodes during the procedure.

## Plasma Vaporization with Button Electrode

The button electrodes are the present day version of vaporization and perhaps nearly replaced all other forms of electrovaporization due to the advantages of being faster and uses of saline irrigation. The movement of the electrode can be much faster than the previous ones, but has to be relatively slow when compared to plasmakinetic resection. The plasma generated all over the button acts to vaporize the tissue. A systematic sequence is followed and tissue vaporized by moving the button electrode over the entire surface of the prostate. At the bladder neck, the direction of the movement can be sideways to achieve smoother surface. Rest of the tissue is vaporized in sequence of choice. The tissue and vessels get vaporized and coagulated and hence the vision remains extremely clear as compared to even plasmakinetic resection. This clear vision translates to compensate for the slower pace of movements. There have been usage of this advantage to perform the procedures in patients using anticoagulants (Fig. 9.30).

To further enhance the pace of vaporization with button electrode, especially in relatively larger glands, there have been modifications in technique. The first one is vaporesection, wherein the button electrode is used to create grooves and resect off small wedges of gland. This process can be further extended into the technique of vapoenucleation. Here the principles of enucleation are followed but the button electrode is used to achieve it. Grooves on roof and bottom of gland are created at 12 o'clock and 6 o'clock respectively. These extend from bladder neck to the distal extent of adenoma. Once grooves are created, the junction of adenoma with mucosa is marked as the distal extent of clearance. The enucleation is begun with vaporization in an attempt to connect the 6 o'clock and 12 o'clock grooves over the entire length of the prostate beginning distally and proceeding toward the bladder neck. Once the two grooves are connected, the lobe will be attached only by a short segment at the bladder neck. It is left attached at this level and the button electrode is changed to a loop and the devascularized lobe resected off. Similar process is performed on both sides either simultaneously or sequentially (Figs. 9.31 to 9.36).

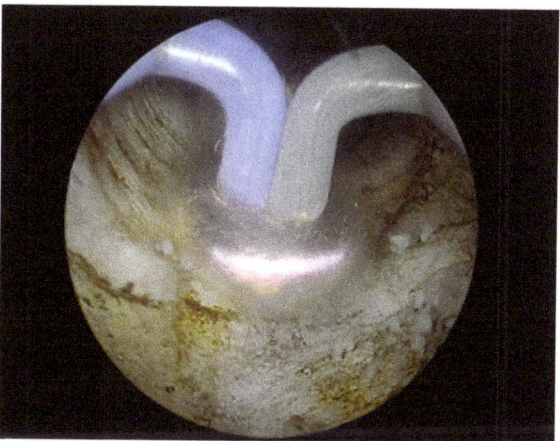

**Fig. 9.30:** Plasma button vaporization.

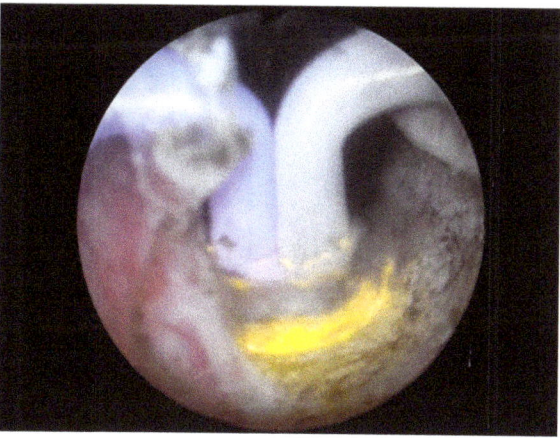

**Fig. 9.31:** Groove on the floor at 7 o'clock position. Similar groove also done at 5 o'clock position.

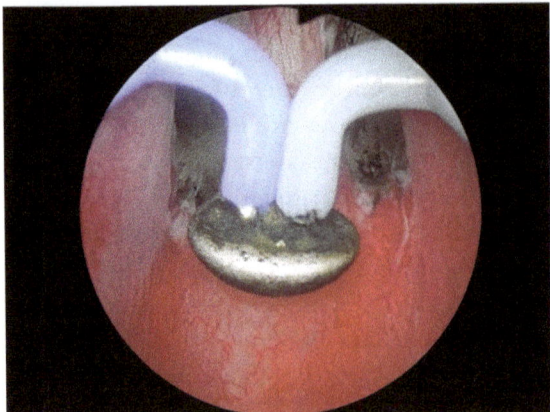

**Fig. 9.32:** The two grooves on either side of median lobe at 5 o'clock and 7 o'clock positions.

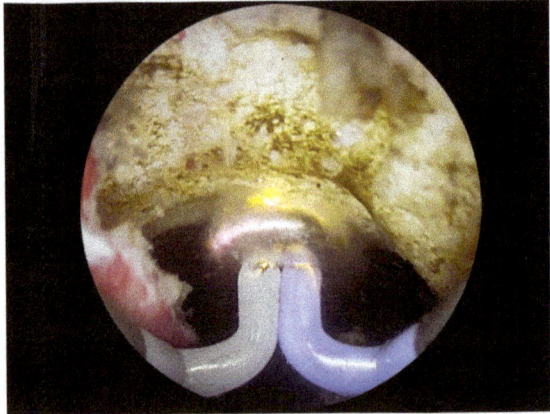

**Fig. 9.33:** Groove on roof at 12 o'clock position.

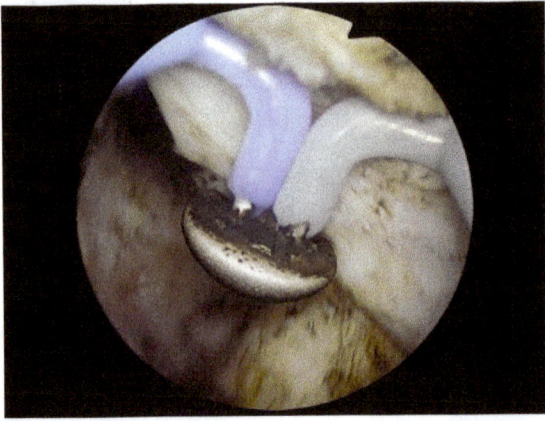

**Fig. 9.34:** Enucleation of the median lobe from the 7 o'clock groove.

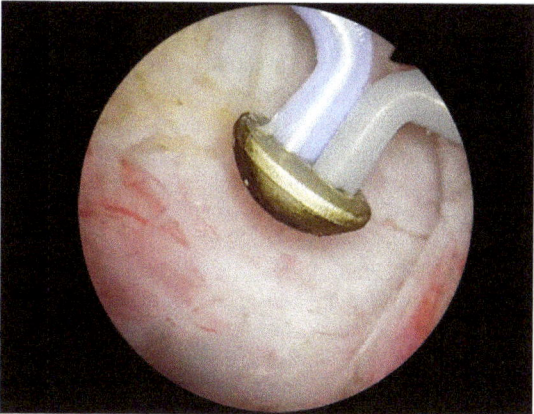

**Fig. 9.35:** Enucleation of right lateral lobe.

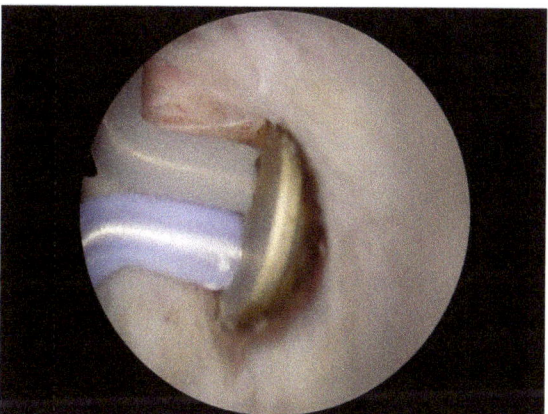

**Fig. 9.36:** Enucleation of the left lateral lobe.

## CONCLUSION

Transurethral vaporization of prostate and TUVRP were based on usage of high power to tissues to achieve vaporization and desiccation. Efficacy was found similar to that of TURP in smaller glands on short-term follow-up. The duration of catheterization was shown to be less and operative time found to be longer. Robust meta-analysis and randomized controlled trials (RCTs) were lacking to make a claim for these as an alternative to TURP. With the advent of plasmakinetic vaporization, the operative times have reduced maintaining the shorter catheterization duration. Plasmakinetic vaporesection and vapo-enucleation attempt to address the issue of larger glands and lack of tissue for histopathology. Meta-analysis found it comparable to bipolar TURP and this may be the contender for a spot close to bipolar TURP for minimally invasive surgical treatment of BPH.

## BIBLIOGRAPHY

1. Aus G, Bergdahl S, Frösing R, et al. Reference range of prostate-specific antigen after transurethral resection of the prostate. Urology. 1996;47:529-31.
2. Cabelin MA, Te AE, Kaplan SA. Transurethral vaporization of the prostate: current techniques. Curr Urol Rep. 2000;1:116-23.
3. Gilling PJ, Kennett K, Das AK, et al. Holmium laser enucleation of the prostate (HoLEP) combined with transurethral tissue morcellation: an update on the early clinical experience. J Endourol. 1998;12:457-9.
4. Gilling PJ, Kennett KM, Fraundorfer MR. Holmium laser enucleation of the prostate for glands larger than 100 g: an endourologic alternative to open prostatectomy. J Endourol. 2000;14:529-31.
5. Kaplan SA, Laor E, Fatal M, et al. Transurethral resection of the prostate versus transurethral electrovaporization of the prostate: a blinded, comparative study with 1-year followup. J Urol. 1998;159:454-8.
6. Kaplan SA, Te AE. Transurethral electrovaporization of the prostate (TVP): a novel method for treating men with benign prostatic hyperplasia. Urology. 1995;45:566-72.
7. Kuntz RM. Current role of lasers in the treatment of benign prostatic hyperplasia (BPH). Eur Urol. 2006;49:961-9.
8. Kuntz RM, Lehrich K, Ahyai SA. Holmium laser enucleation of the prostate versus open prostatectomy for prostates greater than 100 grams: 5-year follow-up results of a randomised clinical trial. Eur Urol. 2008;53:160-6.
9. Küpeli S, Soygür T, Yilmaz E, et al. Combined transurethral resection and vaporization of the prostate using newly designed electrode: a promising treatment alternative for benign prostatic hyperplasia. J Endourol. 1999;13:225-8.
10. Lin Y, Wu X, Xu A, et al. Transurethral enucleation of the prostate versus transvesical open prostatectomy for large benign prostatic hyperplasia: a systematic review and meta-analysis of randomized controlled trials. World J Urol. 2016;34:1207-19.
11. Liu C, Zheng S, Li H, et al. Transurethral enucleation and resection of prostate in patients with benign prostatic hyperplasia by plasma kinetics. J Urol. 2010;184:2440-5.
12. Mauermayer W. Transurethral Surgery. Berlin Heidelberg, New York: Springer-Verlag; 1983.
13. Mebust WK. Transurethral surgery. In: Walsh PC, Retik AB, Vaughn ED Jr, Wein AJ (Eds). Campbell's Urology, 7th edition. Philadelphia: WB Saunders Co; 1998. pp. 1511-28.
14. Mu XN, Wang SJ, Chen J, et al. Bipolar transurethral enucleation of prostate versus photoselective vaporisation for symptomatic benign prostatic hyperplasia (>70 ml). Asian J Androl. 2017;19:608-12.
15. Naspro R, Bachmann A, Gilling P, et al. A review of the recent evidence (2006-2008) for 532-nm photoselective laser vaporisation and holmium laser enucleation of the prostate. Eur Urol. 2009;55:1345-57.
16. Naspro R, Suardi N, Salonia A, et al. Holmium laser enucleation of the prostate versus open prostatectomy for prostates >70 g: 24-month follow-up. Eur Urol. 2006;50:563-8.
17. Neill MG, Gilling PJ, Kennett KM, et al. Randomized trial comparing holmium laser enucleation of prostate with plasmakinetic enucleation of prostate for treatment of benign prostatic hyperplasia. Urology. 2006;68:1020-4.

18. Ou R, Deng X, Yang W, et al. Transurethral enucleation and resection of the prostate vs transvesical prostatectomy for prostate volumes >80 mL: a prospective randomized study. BJU Int. 2013;112:239-45.
19. Perlmutter AP, Muschter R, Razvi HA. Electrosurgical vaporization of the prostate in the canine model. Urology. 1995;46:518-23.
20. Sevryukov FA, Nakagawa K. The Use of Bipolar Transurethral Enucleation for the Treatment of Large-sized Benign Prostatic Hyperplasia. Sovremennye Tehnologii v Medicine. 2012;3:46-8.
21. Stewart S, Benjamin D, Ruckle HC, et al. Electrovaporization of the prostate: new technique for the treatment of symptomatic benign hyperplasia. J Endourol. 1995;9:413-6.
22. Talic RF, El Tiraifi A, El Faqih SR, et al. Prospective randomized study of transurethral vaporization resection of the prostate using the thick loop and standard transurethral prostatectomy. Urology. 2000;55:886-90.
23. van Swol CF, van Vliet RJ, Verdaasdonk RM, et al. Electrovaporization as a treatment modality for transurethral resection of the prostate: influence of generator type. Urology. 1999;53:317-21.
24. Yong Wei, Ning Xu, Shao-Hao Chen, et al. Bipolar transurethral enucleation and resection of the prostate versus bipolar resection of the prostate for prostates larger than 60 gm: A retrospective study at a single academic tertiary care center. Int Braz J Urol. 2016;42:747-56.
25. Zhang KY, Xing JC, Chen BS, et al. Bipolar plasmakinetic transurethral resection of the prostate vs. transurethral enucleation and resection of the prostate: pre- and postoperative comparisons of parameters used in assessing benign prostatic enlargement. Singapore Med J. 2011;52:747-687514.
26. Zhao Z, Zeng G, Zhong W, et al. A prospective, randomised trial comparing plasmakinetic enucleation to standard transurethral resection of the prostate for symptomatic benign prostatic hyperplasia: three-year follow-up results. Eur Urol. 2010;58:752-8.
27. Narayan P, Tewari A, Croker B, et al. Factors affecting size and configuration of electrovaporization lesions in the prostate. Urology. 1996;47(5):679-88.

# Chapter 10

# Laser Enucleation and Vaporization of Prostate

*Arunkumar, R Vijayakumar*

## HISTORICAL BACKGROUND

Holmium laser application for prostate was first reported in 1995 by Gilling et al. Initially it was used for prostate ablation. The Holmium:yttrium-aluminum-garnet (Ho:YAG) laser with a wavelength of 2410 nm is strongly absorbed by water molecules and has a short tissue penetration of 0.5 mm. Hence the tissue needs to be in contact with the laser fiber for effect (contact laser). Tissue vaporization is caused by photothermal effect. The low ablation velocity made it effective only for small prostates of 30 g. Gilling modified this method to resect the prostate tissue into small bits, similar to transurethral resection of the prostate (TURP) [holmium laser resection of the prostate (HoLRP)]. But HoLRP is very much time consuming compared to classical TURP. The main drawback was the time taken for the removal of the resected bits. Fraundorfer and Gilling in 1998 reported prostate enucleation and removal of adenoma with tissue morcellator [holmium laser enucleation of the prostate (HoLEP)]. This procedure has proved to be the best utilization of holmium laser in the management of benign prostatic hyperplasia (BPH).

## PREOPERATIVE WORKUP

General indications, contraindications, and preoperative workup are similar to any other patient with BPH. Patients on anticoagulants and antiplatelets are not contraindicated for HoLEP. But in the initial part of career, it is advisable to take up the patients after stopping antiplatelets and anticoagulants. Even patients on anticoagulants, which could not be withheld can be taken up for HoLEP with caution.

### Equipment

The inner resectoscope sheaths for laser fiber are of two types. The Iglesias type resectoscope with TURP working element mechanism and the other is a bridge for stabilizing the laser fiber. 6- or 7-Fr ureteral catheter is preferred for stabilizing the fiber by some surgeons. Tissue morcellators with normal saline as irrigant are used commonly through 25- to 27-Fr indirect Nephroscopes. A 100 W laser with an end-firing 550 µ laser fiber is preferred. The power settings at the start are typically 2.0 J and 40 Hz is preferred. Lower power lasers (80 or 60 W) will need a comparatively longer duration of resection.

## Preparation for Resection

The initial steps of cystoscopy and introduction of scope and sheath is similar to TURP and described elsewhere in this book. Once the sheath is inserted, the fiber stabilizing catheter is inserted and locked. The laser fiber is threaded through the catheter and approximately 2 cm length of the fiber should be beyond the sheath to prevent damage to the lens. The cystoscopic landmarks are confirmed once again and enucleation is started. If the median lobe is large, it is resected first, else lateral lobe resection is started.

### Enucleation of Median Lobe

The initial landmark to be visualized before median lobe enucleation are the sulci at 5 o'clock and 7 o'clock positions (Fig. 10.1). These form the junction of the median and lateral lobes. Enucleation is started by making a groove in either 5 o'clock or 7 o'clock position with laser, along the sulcus. The groove extends from the bladder neck proximally to verumontanum distally. The distal end is just proximal and lateral to verumontanum.

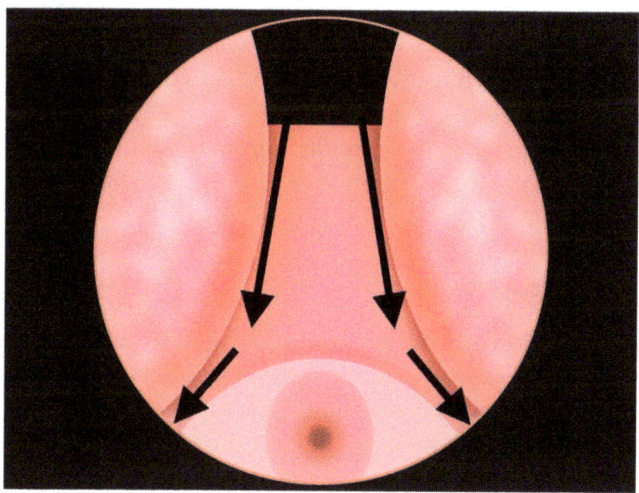

**Fig. 10.1:** Enucleation of median lobe started from 5 o'clock and 7 o'clock positions.

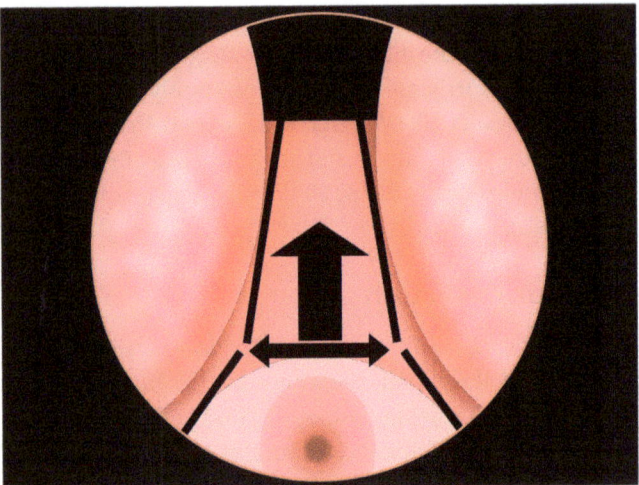

**Fig. 10.2:** Median lobe enucleation completed by connecting the two grooves transversely and lifting it from the capsule.

The groove is deepened to the capsule which is seen as circular pearly white fibers. Capsular fibers are better visualized in the proximal part of prostate. Gradually the groove is widened and undermined to separate the lateral (right or left) and median lobe. The distal margin can be delineated beforehand by creating a groove beneath the lateral lobes, lateral to then verumontanum, so that we do not overshoot the limits and also the depth distally, in the initial cases. Once both grooves are created, they are connected just proximal to verumontanum. The laser fiber is moved transversely along the plane between the adenoma and capsule developed previously, connecting both grooves. As the distal median lobe is gradually getting separated, the capsular plane can be better defined by using the resectoscope beak, to "lever" out the adenoma from the capsule. Capsule appears as glistening white fiber with minimal cobweb like attachments. The separation proceeds proximally *along the curve of the prostate* along the plane of the capsule till the bladder neck. We should make sure we do not undermine the trigone. The median lobe is then freed at the level of bladder neck and pushed into the bladder (Fig. 10.2).

*Lateral Lobe Dissection Initiation*

In those with *absence* of median lobe enlargement, the initial groove is developed at 6 o'clock position and then, the lateral lobe enucleation is started. Once the capsular plane is identified, the adenoma is lifted up using the side-to-side motion of the laser fiber in the capsular plane, assisted by lifting of the adenoma by the beak of the resectoscope. Adequate space for resting the beak of the scope should be ensured before lifting, to prevent

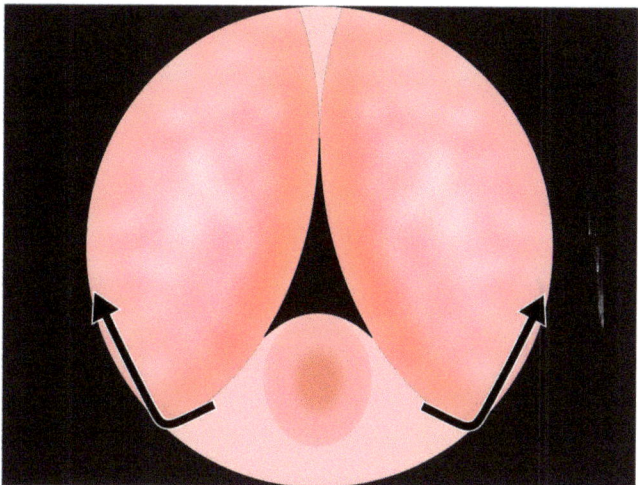

**Fig. 10.3:** Enucleation of the lateral lobes started from the apical part of the lobes close to the sphincter and extending proximally.

the fiber tip accidentally entering the adenoma obscuring the plane. The plane is developed till the bladder neck (Fig. 10.3).

### Lateral and Apical Lobe Dissection

As the enucleation proceeds, some restriction is noted due to the attachments in the lateral and apical aspects. This usually occurs when adenoma is lifted beyond 7 o'clock position. Then the apical and lateral incision is commenced. Scope is withdrawn till verumontanum to assess the apex. Apical tissue is lifted off similarly, extending the incision further laterally and the same plane is developed proximally. Lateral dissection proceeds till 9–10 o'clock position, from apical lobe to bladder neck. The power is 2 J and frequency 30 Hz at the apex to prevent thermal injury. Gradual movement of the resectoscope in the clockwise and anticlockwise motion, along the curvature of the capsule, helps in lifting the adenoma in the same plane. This is continued till the bladder neck (Fig. 10.3).

### Anterior Groove Creation and Separation

Once lateral lobe is dissected till 10 o'clock position, anterior commissure is incised to form a groove at 12 o'clock position (Fig. 10.4). This incision extends from the bladder neck proximally to the level of verumontanum distally. The groove is deepened till capsule. It should be borne in mind that the anterior lobe is thin and capsule is comparatively closer than posterior or lateral aspects. Once the capsule is identified, the groove is extended laterally till the 3 o'clock or 9 o'clock position (Fig. 10.5). The lateral extension of the groove can be started from the verumontanum or the bladder neck.

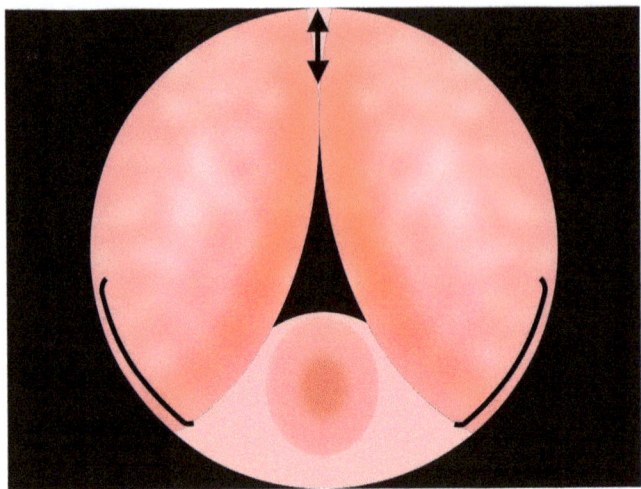

**Fig. 10.4:** Anterior commissure incision at 12 o'clock position, from bladder neck to verumontanum.

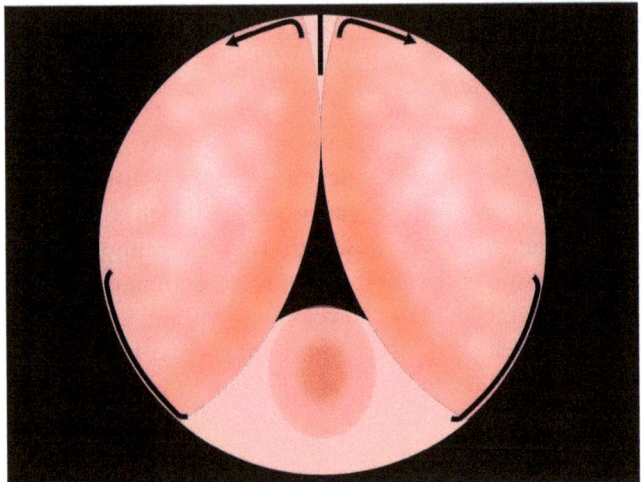

**Fig. 10.5:** Anterior incision extended to 3 o'clock and 9 o'clock position from 12 o'clock position, from the level of verumontanum, till capsule is identified.

### Separation of Lateral Lobe from Roof

The anteriorly developed plane is extended laterally. The anteriorly developing plane and posterior plane may not be exact in many instances. It is better to cross check the posteriorly developed plane intermittently while incising anteriorly. When both incisions are considerably close laterally, the intervening mucosal/fibrous strip is incised and the attachments are freed laterally till the bladder neck. This leaves the lobe attached only by a band

# Laser Enucleation and Vaporization of Prostate

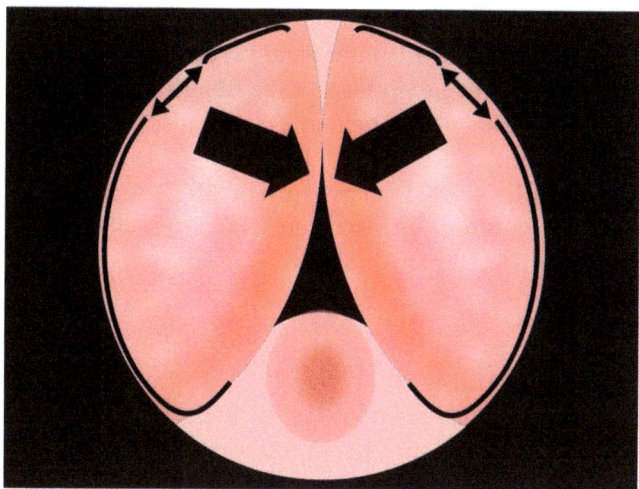

**Fig. 10.6:** Joining both incisions so that the adenoma is lifted up for visualization of stalk.

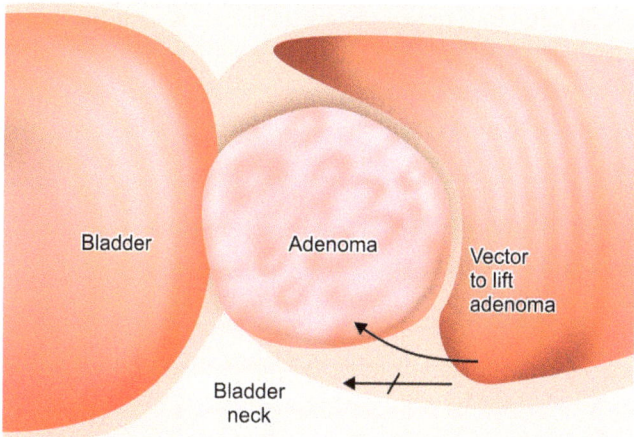

**Fig. 10.7:** Lifting of adenoma to visualize the stalk at the level of bladder neck.

of tissue at the bladder neck. This part is approached from beneath the adenoma and incised. Undermining the bladder neck is a possibility at this juncture and it should be carefully avoided. The freed adenoma is pushed into the bladder (Fig. 10.6 and 10.7).

Contralateral lobe enucleation is carried out similarly and all the three lobes are placed within the bladder.

## Hemostasis

Coagulation depth of Ho:YAG laser is 3-4 mm. Since tissue morcellation needs clear vision, good hemostasis is essential. Even small bleeders need to be controlled. Two types of vessels have been described in prostate—(1) end vessels (perforating the adenoma) and (2) creeping vessels (network at the level of capsule). For hemostasis, laser should be defocused by firing at an angle. The fiber should be held at 2-3 mm distance from the bleeder. Altering the power to 1.0-1.5 J and 30 Hz may provide better hemostasis of small bleeders. 2.0 J and 30 Hz may be useful for large bleeders.

The whole prostatic fossa is inspected before morcellation. Bleeders are coagulated and residual adenoma if any are vaporized.

### Morcellation

The rigid offset nephroscope may be inserted *through* the outer sheath after removing the inner sheath and laser fiber. Else, the sheath can be removed completely and nephroscope inserted. Dual inflow of irrigant is preferable, through both nephroscope and outer sheath is preferable to ensure distended bladder. Irrigation pump is also useful. Bladder distension is crucial, since partially collapsed bladder can result in bladder injury. The morcellator tip is placed beneath the adenoma and slight suction is applied. As the adenoma attaches to the tip, morcellation is activated and adenoma is shredded. The morcellator tip should be under vision always and away from the bladder wall.

If hard nodules are present in the adenoma, they can be managed with alligator forceps. Smaller bits are removed with Ellick's or Toomey evacuators. In some cases, adenoma can be incised using laser into multiple bits and removed. Mauermayer stone punch may be used at times.

In case of excess bleeding obscuring vision and morcellation, patient is catheterized and taken up for morcellation after 48-72 hours, once urine is clear.

Duration of catheterization after the procedure is 48-72 hours.

## CONCLUSION

Holmium laser enucleation of the prostate is a proven safe and effective procedure. This procedure is akin to simple prostatectomy—adenoma enucleation. 50-60 g prostate is ideal for beginners.

## BIBLIOGRAPHY

1. Descazeaud A, Robert G, Azzousi AR, et al. Laser treatment of benign prostatic hyperplasia in patients on oral anticoagulant therapy: a review. BJU Int. 2009;103:1162-5.
2. Fraundorfer MR, Gilling PJ. Holmium:YAG laser enucleation of the prostate combined with mechanical morcellation: preliminary results Eur Urol. 1998;33:69-72.

3. Gilling PJ, Cass CB, Cresswell MD, et al. Holmium laser resection of the prostate: preliminary results of a new method for the treatment of benign prostatic hyperplasia. Urology. 1996;47:48-51.
4. Gilling PJ, Cass CB, Malcolm AR, et al. Combination holmium and Nd:YAG laser ablation of the prostate: initial clinical experience. J Endourol. 1995;9:151-3.
5. Gilling PJ, Mackey M, Cresswell M, et al. Holmium laser versus transurethral resection of the prostate: a randomized prospective trial with 1-year follow-up. J Urol. 1999;162:1640-4.
6. Krambeck AE, Handa SE, Lingeman JE. Experience with more than 1,000 holmium laser prostate enucleations for benign prostatic hyperplasia. J Urol. 2013;189:S141-5.
7. Kuntz RM, Lehrich K, Ahyai S. Does perioperative outcome of transurethral holmium laser enucleation of the prostate depend on prostate size? J Endourol. 2004;18:183-8.
8. Kuo RL, Paterson RF, Kim SC, et al. Holmium laser enucleation of the prostate (HoLEP): a technical update. World J Surg Oncol. 2003;1:6.
9. Madersbacher S, Alivizatos G, Nordling J, et al. EAU 2004 guidelines on assessment, therapy and follow-up of men with lower urinary tract symptoms suggestive of benign prostatic obstruction (BPH guidelines). Eur Urol. 2004;46:547-54.
10. McVary KT, Roehrborn CG, Avins AL, et al. Update on AUA guideline on the management of benign prostatic hyperplasia. J Urol. 2011;185:1793-803.
11. Shah HN, Mahajan AP, Hegde SS, et al. Perioperative complications of holmium laser enucleation of the prostate: experience in the first 280 patients, and a review of literature. BJU Int. 2007;100:94-101.
12. Tan AH, Gilling PJ. Holmium laser prostatectomy: current techniques. Urology. 2002;60:152-6.

# Chapter 11

# Transurethral Resection of Bladder Tumor

*RM Meyyappan*

## INTRODUCTION

Urothelial carcinoma is the most common malignancy of the urinary tract and is the second most common cause of death among genitourinary tumors. Transurethral resection of bladder tumor (TURBT) is both diagnostic (evaluation of tumor stage and grade) and therapeutic (for nonmuscle invasive tumors) for bladder tumors.

## CARCINOMA BLADDER

Urothelial cancer is a disease of the aged, with a peak in the eighth decade of life. Its incidence has a strong association with environmental toxins. The incidence rate has been rising over the last 60–70 years. Smoking is one of the primary causes, in addition to genetic abnormalities, carcinogen exposure, nutritional factors, alcohol, inflammation, infection, chemotherapy, radiation, and possibly artificial sweeteners. Gross, painless hematuria is the primary symptom in 85% of patients with a newly diagnosed bladder tumor, and microscopic hematuria occurs in virtually all patients.

Histologically, 90% of bladder cancers are transitional cell carcinomas, 5% are squamous cell carcinomas, and less than 2% are adenocarcinoma or other variants. At initial presentation, 80% of urothelial tumors are nonmuscle invasive. Their physical appearance varies from polypoid papillary tumors (low or high grade) and sessile solid growths (mostly high grade) to "flat" carcinoma in situ (CIS) lesions.

## EVALUATION

Cystoscopy, upper tract imaging (contrast CT with urogram), and urine cytology are necessary in the evaluation of carcinoma bladder. Upper tract imaging is usually performed before transurethral resection (TUR) both to identify other sources of hematuria and to assess the extravesical urothelium because of the "field change" nature of UC, which can affect such tissue throughout the urinary tract. NMP22 tumor markers may be used in select cases.

## TRANSURETHRAL RESECTION OF BLADDER TUMOR PROCEDURE

Transurethral resection of bladder tumor under regional or general anesthesia is the initial treatment for visible lesions. The objectives of TURBT are:
- To remove all visible tumors
- To provide specimens for pathologic examination to accurately determine stage and grade.

The information from TURBT should answer the following questions:
- Whether it is a palpable mass and whether it is mobile.
- Tumor characters—configuration (papillary versus solid), location, extent (bladder neck and urethra), number, and size
- Presence of carcinoma in situ
- Quality of resection—complete/incomplete
- Deep biopsy from the tumor bed.

The answers to all the questions should be available in the operation notes of TURBT.

## SURGICAL INSTRUMENTATION

The equipment used for TURBT is nearly identical to that used for transurethral resection of the prostate (TURP):
- Endoscopic sheaths (e.g. 20 Fr, 24 Fr, 27 Fr, and deflecting sheaths) with their respective obturators.
- Resecting loops (24 Fr and 27 Fr loop, rolling ball, and right-angle electrodes).
- Marberger cold-cup biopsy forceps.
- Diathermy generator with grounding pad
- Lenses (30° and 70° lenses with spares)
- Irrigation tubing and irrigant, water-soluble lubricant, urethral sounds, light source with camera.
- Evacuators (Toomey, Ellik, or Creevy) with specimen cups and labels are needed.
- Numerous urethral catheters should be on hand for post-procedure bladder drainage including conventional Foley and Coudé catheters as well as three-way catheters for continuous bladder irrigation [Continuous bladder irrigation (CBI) or Murphy drip].

Based on the information available (preoperative cystoscopy/CT), adjustments in equipment selection and technique may be needed.

## IRRIGATING SOLUTIONS

Since the bladder does not readily absorb its contents, the use of sterile water is safe, is unlikely to result in hemolysis or hyponatremia [TUR syndrome (TURS)], and yields outstanding endoscopic visualization. Else, glycine is the usual preferred alternative. For bipolar TURBT, normal saline solution is used as the irrigant. The various irrigants used and their advantages and disadvantages are discussed elsewhere in this book.

## SURGICAL APPROACH

Transurethral resection of bladder tumor starts with bimanual (bidigital) examination of the bladder. It is usually done after anesthesia, before draping. It reveals the palpability and fixity of the tumor. It is repeated after TURBT also, to find out any change in the findings.

### Initial Cystoscopy

White light cystoscopy (WLC) is the gold standard for initial evaluation. Flexible office cystoscopy is as reliable as rigid endoscopy *for evaluation* and has excellent sensitivity and specificity for papillary tumors but is relatively poor for CIS. Complete visualization to plan the resection is facilitated by either the flexible cystoscope or preferably the 70° rigid rod lens.

Fluorescence cystoscopy uses photoactive porphyrins (hexaminolevulinate) that accumulate preferentially in neoplastic tissue and emit red fluorescence under blue-wavelength light. This may improve the detection of small papillary lesions and CIS. Narrow-band imaging (NBI) is an endoscopic optical image enhancement technique that enhances the contrast between mucosal surfaces and microvascular structures without the use of dyes. These are not essential for TURBT, but helpful in ensuring complete resection, if available.

*Resection*: Resection is performed using a 30° lens placed through a resectoscope sheath. This lens angulation allows visualization of the loop during resection. Continuous irrigation, with a partially filled bladder (filled enough to visualize bladder contents) minimizes bladder wall movement prevents stretching of detrusor and its thinning. This decreases the risk of perforation.

Resection is performed piecemeal in most of the cases. Small tumors can be removed en bloc. It is advisable to start the resection *from the edge of the tumor*, if piecemeal excision is planned. This is helpful since the main vascularity is from the center, containing larger vessels. Vascularity is lesser in the edges and hemostasis and visibility is better when the more vascular central part of the tumor is resected. In larger tumors, retaining the stalk or stem portion in the initial part of resection of the tumor helps to maintain counter traction and makes resection easier. Once the majority of the tumor is resected, the stalk can be excised along with remaining tumor. In large tumors with overhanging edges, lifting the tumor edge with the loop, away from the bladder, lessens the chance of perforation (Figs. 11.1 and 11.2).

In case of smaller tumors, single pass resection of the tumor along its base is feasible (Figs. 11.3A to D). It should not be attempted for larger tumors (larger than those removable through the sheath). Then, they need some mechanical morcellation to remove through the sheath. This may become a cumbersome process at the end.

Friable, low-grade tumors can often be removed without the use of electrical energy. The tumor is fragmented by the "mechanical force" of the loop. The bleeders opened may be coagulated. This minimizes the chance of bladder perforation and unnecessary diathermy damage or loss of specimens.

Many tumors extend 1–2 cm beyond the visible margin of the polyp. Hence, it is advisable to extend the margin of resection 1–2 cm beyond the visible lesion.

Higher-grade, solid tumors and the base of all tumors require the use of diathermy, cutting current. This helps in precise resection of tissues. After all the visible tumor has been resected, an additional pass of the cutting loop or a cold-cup biopsy from the tumor base, including the muscle, should be obtained to send to pathology separately. This is essential to confirm muscle invasion. A chip evacuator gathers the specimen. Final confirmation of hemostasis in the presence of minimal irrigation after all chips have been removed through vigorous irrigation is necessary. The tumor bed has to be in perfect hemostasis with the use of coagulating current and preferably "roller ball" electrode.

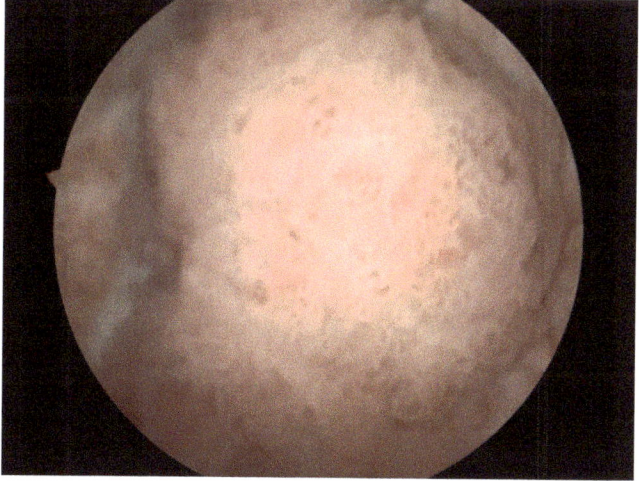

**Fig. 11.1:** Large bladder tumor which needs piecemeal excision.

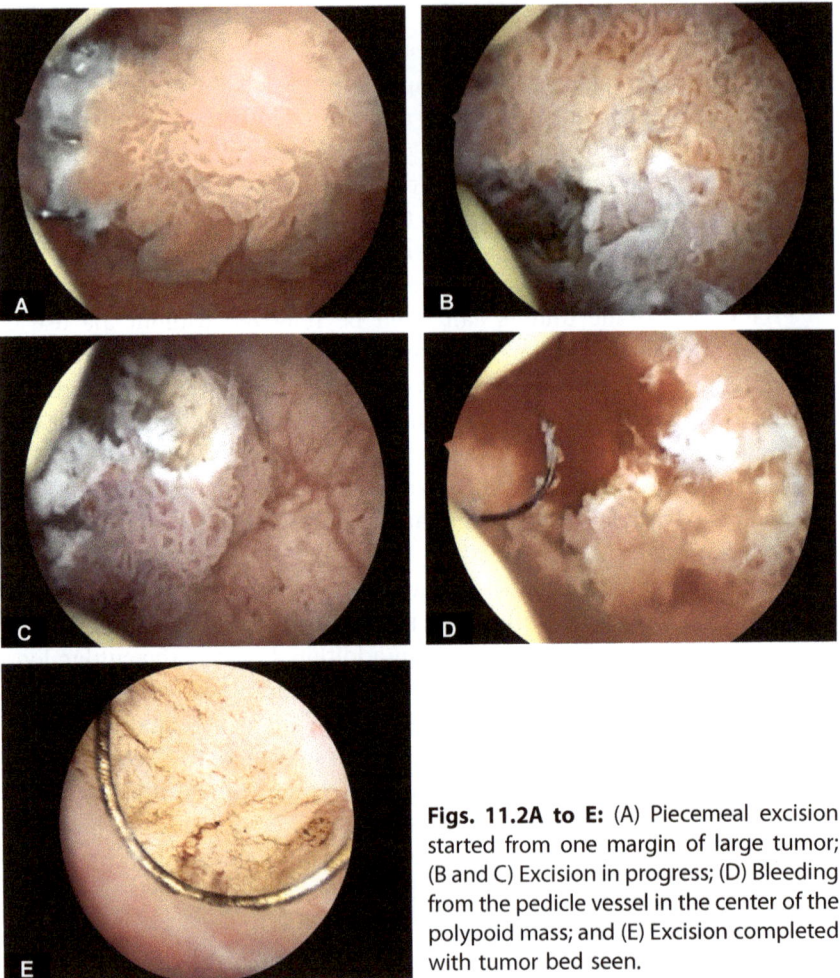

**Figs. 11.2A to E:** (A) Piecemeal excision started from one margin of large tumor; (B and C) Excision in progress; (D) Bleeding from the pedicle vessel in the center of the polypoid mass; and (E) Excision completed with tumor bed seen.

Random bladder biopsies are recommended to detect unsuspected CIS or small papillary tumors in endoscopically normal urothelium. This is especially necessary, if the cytology is high grade tumor and all the tumors in the bladder appear to be low grade and polypoid.

## Diffuse Carcinoma In Situ

If carcinoma *in situ* changes (diffuse velvety erythematous areas) involves small areas of the bladder, biopsies are done and lesions fulgurated. If extensive areas are involved, random biopsies and follow up with intravesical BCG is preferable. Electric desiccation of large areas of bladder mucosa can cause bladder contracture.

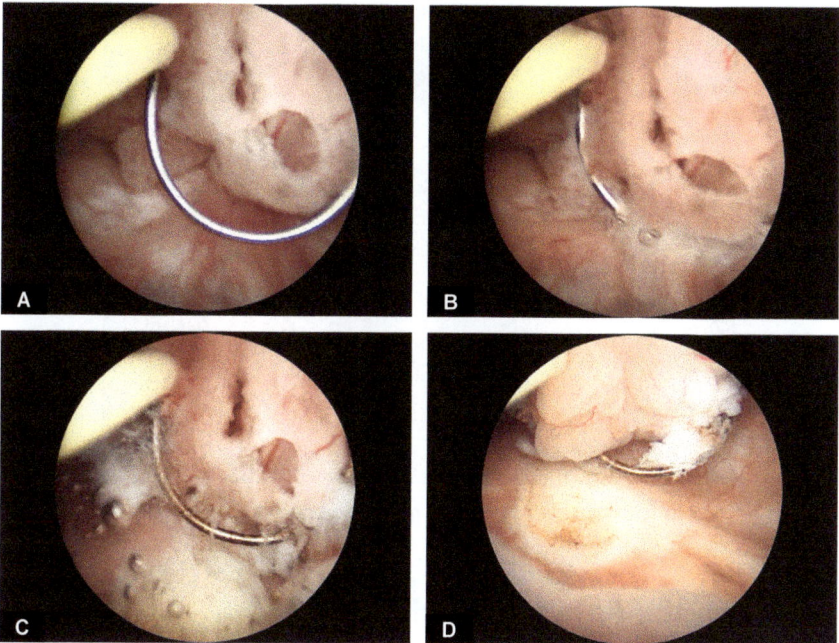

**Figs. 11.3A to D:** (A) Small tumor amenable for en bloc excision; (B and C) Excision in progress; and (D) Excision completed.

## Tumor Involving the Ureteral Orifice

These kinds of tumors need special care during resection. There should be no compromise on tumor clearance, hemostasis or ureteric lumen. The ureteric orifice can be resected along with the tumor if necessary, for complete clearance. Pure cutting current should be used for resection. Precise coagulation of the bleeders with Collin's knife tip or Bugbee electrode aids in preventing stricture.

Stenting helps in preventing stricture in some cases. If the tumor is close to the orifice and the orifice is visible, stenting prior to resection is advisable. In the event of resection of ureteric orifice, pink fluffy mucosa of the ureter can be identified in the pearly white tumor bed (Fig. 11.4).

If the orifice is still not visible, intravenous methylene blue instillation can be done to see the efflux. The other option is to conclude the procedure and plan for percutaneous nephrostomy if the patient develops flank pain with hydronephrosis. Most often there is no need for intervention if pure cutting current alone was used at resection.

Tumor location at the ureteral orifice should not deter appropriate endoscopic management. Reflux of urine into the upper tracts may occur with ureteral stenting or through vesicoureteral reflux following resection of the ureteral orifice. Its significance in risk to tumor seeding in upper tract is controversial.

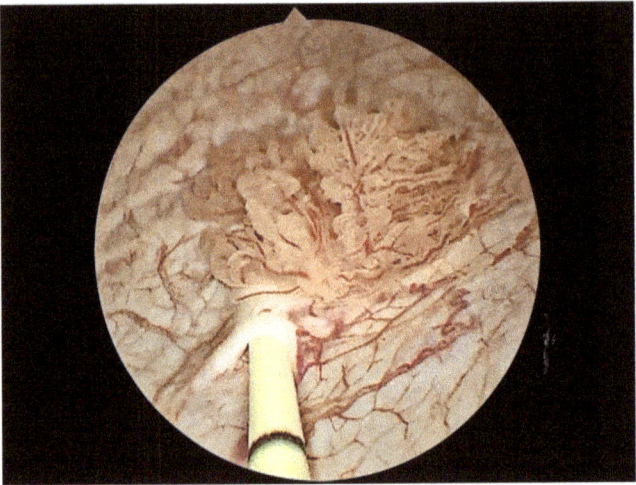

**Fig. 11.4:** Ureteric catheter *in situ* while resecting tumors close to ureteric orifice.

## Tumor on the Anterior Bladder Wall

Anterior bladder wall tumor resection is done with 30° scope inverted upside down. Resection is facilitated by applying downward suprapubic pressure (compressing the anterior wall toward the posterior wall) with the non-dominant hand. The bladder should be only partially filled with irrigant to allow better visualization of the tumor.

## Tumor at the Dome

Resection at the bladder dome is challenging because of its anatomic relationships. Since the bladder dome is the furthest point from the trigone, visualization is difficult. More irrigant is used to clear away blood, causing the point of interest to travel farther from the resectoscope. A continuous flow resectoscope sheath can be especially useful in this situation. Additionally, bowel can overly the dome and be injured by transmural current from aggressive electrocautery. Finally, elderly patients in general and postmenopausal women in particular have significantly thinner bladder walls; therefore, perforation is an even greater concern in these patients. Taking care not to overdistend the bladder and paying meticulous attention to resection technique and depth are important when working at the bladder dome.

## Tumor at the Lateral Wall

Obturator jerk and the resultant bladder perforation is one of the worrisome complication associated with lateral wall tumors. The obturator nerves

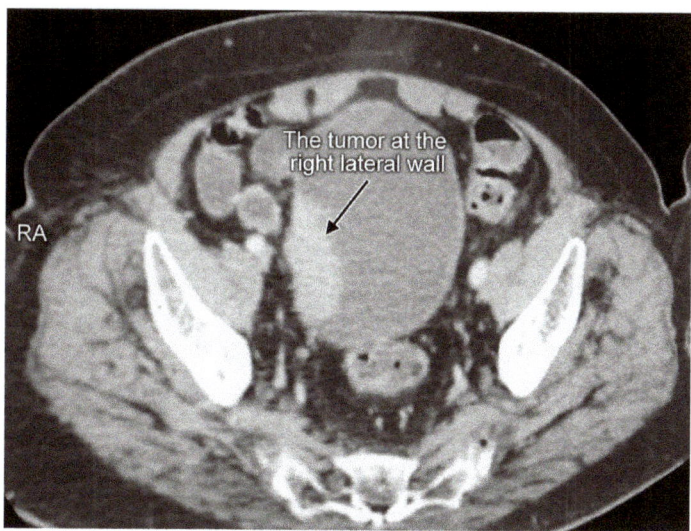

**Fig. 11.5:** Computed tomography (CT) image of tumor in lateral wall of bladder—this tumor needs obturator block to prevent obturator jerk.

course along the lateral pelvic wall in the true pelvis. Bladder distension results in close apposition of the bladder wall to the nerve. Applying diathermy in the lateral wall, results in direct transmission of current to the nerve through the detrusor. The nerve is stimulated and the adductor muscles contract. This sudden jerky movement may cause deeper cut and perforation of bladder (Fig. 11.5).

Preventing overdistension, decreasing the cutting or coagulation current settings, and using intermittent cautery can lessen the incidence of adductor contraction. Injecting local anesthetic directly into the base of the tumor can also have an effect of block, if classical obturator block is not given already. Albeit not foolproof, use of a bipolar resecting system may decrease the incidence of obturator jerk.

## Tumor in Bladder Diverticulum

Bladder diverticulum is the mucosal outpouching, which lacks muscularis propria. This feature renders them thinner and more prone to perforation. This characteristic can also complicate the pathologic staging of lesions within diverticula. Tumor extension beyond the mucosa is akin to T3 (extravesical extension). Hence, "complete" resection results in perforation. Resection of all visible tumor and follow up may be feasible in highly compliant patients. Else, partial cystectomy is the alternative.

## Reducing Cautery Artifact

Excessive cautery artifact is both counterproductive and preventable. Cold-cup biopsies can be obtained before resection or fulguration. Using the lowest and most effective diathermy settings and preferential use of cutting current help in decreasing the artifacts. Use of bipolar energy has not been shown to decrease the degree of cautery artifact. Excessively slow movement of the cautery loop can char the tissue and prevent clean cutting. As such, initiation of the cautery pedal before tissue contact, and swift, controlled movement of the loop through the tissue will maximize specimen preservation.

## Bipolar Energy

Bipolar diathermy is now used in some centers for TURBT. The potential benefits are decreased risk of bladder perforation from obturator reflex and decreased risk of TURS. The technique of TURBT is essentially same. Using saline as irrigant may decrease hemolysis and vision is slightly poorer than the monopolar diathermy with water or glycine as an irrigant.

## Use of Lasers

Different types of lasers have been evaluated as alternative for monopolar TURBT, including neodymium:yttrium-aluminum-garnet (Nd:YAG), argon, potassium titanyl phosphate (KTP), and holmium:YAG. The Nd:YAG laser and Ho:YAG lasers have been found to be useful. The lasers can be used for both ablation and "resection" too. KTP laser is only used for tumor ablation. Since we need specimen for pathological examination, cold cup biopsies need to be performed prior to ablation. With YAG lasers, both resection and ablation can be done. For small tumors, base of the tumor pedicle is lased and the lesion is excised completely. For larger tumors, combined ablation and resection akin to classical TURBT provides specimen for examination and also better hemostasis. Determining tumor depth or muscular invasion may not be readily possible with this type of resection; hence, laser TURBT is mainly preferred for recurrent papillary low-grade tumors. The most significant complication of laser use is the transmural passage of energy resulting in the perforation of an adjacent structure such as an overlying loop of bowel, but this risk is low since the depth of penetration of laser energy is minimal (0.5-3 mm; varying between different types of lasers).

*Post-procedure care*: Insertion of a transurethral catheter is common after TURBT. Choosing a three-way (20-24 Fr) catheter enables the use of continuous bladder irrigation, (CBI or Murphy drip) in the recovery room, if needed. It is critical to include orders for scheduled and as needed manual irrigation with 60-120 mL of normal saline through a 60 mL catheter-tipped syringe to remove any sediment or small blood clots that may have formed.

Catheter block with irrigation in flow can result in bladder rupture, if not detected and relieved early. CBI should be gravity fed only. CBI is contraindicated in patients with bladder perforation. Titrating the flow of pink urine is usually adequate to limit clot formation.

*Postoperative mitomycin C*: Evidence strongly supports the benefit of intravesical mitomycin C immediately after TURBT, in preventing recurrence. The absolute contraindications for intravesical instillation are bladder perforation, allergic reactions to mitomycin and gross hematuria. The instillation is preferable within 6 hours of TURBT. The benefit is negligible or nil if it is given after 24 hours. After TURBT, once the urine appears clear *without irrigation*, 40 mg of mitomycin C is diluted in 20–40 mL of saline and instilled into the bladder. The catheter is clamped for a holding period of 60 min, and the catheter is unclamped.

## COMPLICATIONS OF TRANSURETHRAL RESECTION OF BLADDER TUMORS AND MANAGEMENT

### Overall Morbidity and Mortality

Although TURBT is typically a safe and well-tolerated procedure, urologists must be mindful of the morbidity (5.1–43.3%) and mortality rates (0.8–1.3%) reported in the literature.

### Postoperative Bleeding

Postoperative bleeding is the most frequently reported complication of TURBT; rates range from 2% to 13%. Intraoperative or postoperative bleeding is typically associated with large tumors and extensive or complex resections. Careful examination of all resected areas under little to moderate distension is important to avoid missing small vessels temporarily tamponaded by a distended bladder. Unfortunately, coughing by the patient on emergence from general anesthesia can cause a significant increase in blood pressure resulting in opening up of plugged blood vessels.

The clots forming after the bleed are more sinister compared to actual venous oozing. If gross persistent hematuria is seen with recurrent clot obstruction, cystoscopy, clot evacuation, and fulguration is advisable. Presence of pulsatile (waxing and waning) hematuria or sudden massive hematuria indicates active arterial bleed. Such patients are better served by early cystoscopy and fulguration.

### Bladder Perforation (Fig. 11.6)

Bladder perforation can result in numerous sequelae including hemorrhage, TURS, infection, the need for urgent open surgery, tumor

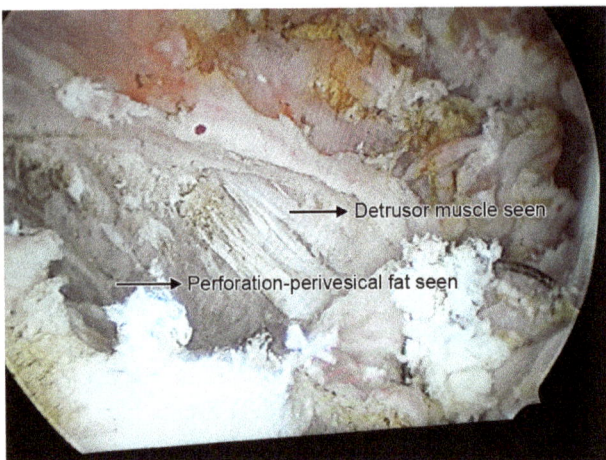

**Fig. 11.6:** Minimal bladder perforation.

spillage, peritonitis, and death. Bladder perforation typically occurs extraperitoneally. This complication can usually be managed with drainage through a urethral catheter, although intraperitoneal rupture is possible and often requires surgical repair (open or laparoscopic). Injuries in the anterior bladder wall, dome, or high posterior wall necessitate a cystogram to rule out intraperitoneal extravasation. Abdominal distension or signs of diaphragmatic irritation during resection may warrant a cystogram or immediate laparotomy, based on the index of suspicion.

If small exposed areas of perivesical fat are observed during resection, without an obvious extravesical pocket or plane, prompt completion of the procedure and placement of a large bore catheter may be sufficient without a cystogram. The incidence of post-TURBT perforations may be underestimated. Balbay and colleagues found contrast extravasation during cystography in 58.3% of their patients, compared with other series reporting perforation in only 1–5% of cases. The significance of these subclinical perforations detected by cystography is unclear.

Although rare, it seems plausible that perforation during TURBT can lead to extravesical disease, which carries a dismal prognosis. It is unclear whether perforation should prompt consideration of systemic treatment in an attempt to mitigate any increased risk of soft tissue seeding. Additionally, the use of perioperative intravesical chemotherapy is contraindicated in the presence of bladder perforation.

## Transurethral Resection Syndrome

Post-TURBT hyponatremia is usually the result of bladder perforation and extravasation or extravesical absorption of irrigant fluid, in contrast to absorption across open prostatic venous sinuses during TURP. Because the irrigant is not directly introduced into the patient's circulatory system and must be absorbed across the peritoneum, the initial presentation may be delayed.

Dorota and colleagues reported a case series of four such events and noted that the time to serum sodium nadir was 2-9 hours, compared with of 1-6 hours following prostatic resection. The signs, symptoms, and management of TURS are described elsewhere in this book.

In addition, bladder perforation has to be ruled out and necessary interventions undertaken if present.

## Infection

Dysuria is common after transurethral bladder surgery, thus patients may have difficulty differentiating the expected symptoms from infection. Similarly, a dipstick urine analysis is difficult to interpret. A short course of postoperative prophylaxis with oral antibiotics is reasonable until the bladder mucosa has had an opportunity to heal. Urine culture is essential and sensitive antibiotics should be started, if culture shows bacterial growth.

## Urinary Retention

Instrumentation, anesthesia (general, spinal, or epidural), and postoperative medicines like narcotic analgesics can precipitate acute urinary retention after catheter removal, especially in men with prostate enlargement. The management involves trial of void undercover of alpha blockers with $5\alpha$-reductase inhibitors. If unsuccessful, TURP is indicated. In those patients on medical management for preexisting BPH with persistent symptoms, TURP can be combined with TURBT. Several studies indicate no change in the disease course, if both procedures are combined.

Urinary retention that occurs weeks to months after TURBT should be investigated with cystoscopy to evaluate for urethral stricture, bladder neck contracture, or tumor recurrence and should be managed appropriately.

# Second Transurethral Resection of Bladder Tumor

A second TURBT, also known as re-staging TURBT, should be considered standard for any high grade tumor, multifocal tumors, the majority of T1 tumors, incompletely resected tumors and if no muscularis propria is identified in the specimens of patients with NMIBC. It is critical to resect all visible papillary tumors, especially T1 lesions, as intravesical BCG is used to treat CIS and does not treat residual papillary tumors.

## RECENT ADVANCES

Local microwave thermotherapy is used with or without combined chemotherapy has been used for surgically unfit candidates with bladder TCC. High intensity focused ultrasound (HIFU), which is more often used in carcinoma prostate, has been used with and without combined intravesical chemotherapy to treat bladder cancer. The combination of mitomycin C and HIFU was felt to be synergistic in indulging tumor necrosis, compared with HIFU alone. The effect of HIFU on the tumor is mainly mediated by thermal energy.

High energy shock waves (HESW), similar to those used for ESWL, and cyberknife are in the experimental stages for treating carcinoma bladder in surgically unfit patients.

# Chapter 12

# Bipolar Transurethral Resection of the Prostate

*Narmada P Gupta, Deepak Rathi*

## INTRODUCTION

Transurethral resection of the prostate (TURP) has become the preferred modality of surgical treatment for benign prostatic hyperplasia (BPH) now. Since its inception, it has undergone several modifications in order to minimize complications and improve results. Bipolar TURP (B-TURP) is one of such modification. In this chapter we shall describe the current status of B-TURP.

## HISTORY OF PROSTATE SURGERY

The first major breakthrough in transurethral surgery was brought in by Hugh Hampton Young in 1909, who invented prostatic punch. In 1926, Maximilian Stern introduced his resectoscope with a tungsten wire loop, which was able to cut "spaghetti-like" pieces of prostate under water. The modern resectoscope, which had a two-handed rack-and-pinion working element was invented by Joseph F McCarthy in 1932. With this resectoscope, loop could be pulled backward away from the bladder neck toward the user. Stern-Davis-McCarthy resectoscope was modified by Reed Nesbit in 1939, who added spring to it and it was made possible to use it single handedly. First successful continuous-flow resectoscope was reported by Iglesias in year 1975.

*Bipolar TURP*: Bipolar TURP overcomes one of the major limitation of monopolar TURP (M-TURP) by allowing resection in normal saline (a conductive fluid medium).

*Mechanism of bipolar TURP*: The Difference in the mechanism of monopolar and bipolar diathermy is explained in detail elsewhere in the book. In short, both the active and neutral leads are in the same electrode. Hence energy is concentrated in the prostate alone, between the two leads. Depth of penetration to surrounding structures is 0.5–1 mm, as compared to 3–5 mm in monopolar.

Energy from bipolar loop do not travel through the body (circuit is complete locally). The energy is transmitted to normal saline and water evaporates creating a gas layer around the loop. This causes excitation of sodium ions, forming plasma, which is a highly energized state of matter around the active electrode consisting of freely moving charged particles (characteristic yellow glow). Plasma causes tissue disruption at molecular level and molecules are cleaved (Flowchart 12.1).

Prostatic tissue removal is similar to M-TURP following the same operative steps. However in contrast to the higher energies used in monopolar resection, B-TURP requires less energy and voltage because there is a smaller amount of interpolated tissue. This lower level of voltage and temperature leads to the reduction of carbonization and of tissue necrosis. In bipolar technique, cutting and coagulation are virtually simultaneous (cut and seal effect of plasma) and these represent concurrent processes. However, for this it is necessary to reduce the speed with which the loop passes through the tissue.

*Comparison of monopolar and bipolar TURP*: Monopolar TURP has been the standard of care, bipolar TURP is one alternative to it, which has been thoroughly investigated. In randomized controlled trials (RCTs) with a follow-up of up to 5 years, no differences were found in efficacy parameters like IPSS, quality of life score and Qmax). Conclusion of all these trials is that B-TURP has equivalent efficacy to M-TURP.

**Flowchart 12.1:** Mechanism of bipolar resection of prostatic tissue.

```
Energy from bipolar loop do not travel through the
body (circuit is complete locally)
            ↓
Energy is transmitted to normal saline
            ↓
Water evaporates creating a gas layer around the loop
            ↓
Excitation of sodium ions
            ↓
These form plasma, a highly energized state of
matter around the active electrode
            ↓
Consisting of freely moving charged particles
(characteristic yellow glow)
            ↓
Plasma causes tissue disruption at molecular level
and molecules are cleaved
```

## COMPLICATIONS

There are no differences in short-term (up to 12 months) urethral stricture and bladder neck contracture rates. A RCT evaluating erectile function showed that both have a similar effect on erectile function. But B-TURP is preferable due to a more favorable perioperative safety profile which includes:

- *Elimination of TUR-syndrome*: One of the major advantages of B-TURP is that issues relating to hypotonic fluid irrigation especially dilutional hyponatremia is eliminated. Use of physiological normal saline for irrigation has practically eliminated it. However, there is risk of fluid absorption through capsular perforations. So one has to be cautious as it can lead to fluid overload, especially in cardiac patients.
- *Allows longer periods of resection*: B-TURP allows for longer resections and meticulous coagulations without the risk of hyponatremia or TUR syndrome. In institutes with residents training programs, it can lead to relaxed training without compromising safety and minimizing patient morbidity.
- *Lower clot retention and lower blood transfusion rates*: With an increase in the elderly on chronic anticoagulation and antiplatelet medications for cardiovascular diseases, there is a greater concern for bleeding. Hemostatic properties of bipolar have been reported to be superior in a number of ex vivo studies. In B-TURP, bleeding occurs at a much lower rate as compared to monopolar and this can be explained by the cut and seal effect of plasma, especially if resection is done slowly. However, more RCTs are needed to clarify which provide better hemostasis.
- *Shorter irrigation and catheterization period and possibly shorter hospitalization times*: Bipolar resection was found in studies superior to monopolar, regarding the reduction of the hemoglobin level (1.2 g/dL vs 1.7 g/dL) and the amount of fluid used for postoperative lavage. Most studies report a decrease of postoperative catheterization period for bipolar technique.
- *Bipolar TURP for large adenomas*: Studies have concluded that B-TURP is an effective and safe alternative to M-TURP in treating patients with large prostates [mean prostate volume (PV) > 70 mL], with the potential of having less perioperative and similar short-term complication rates up to 36 months of follow-up. This is due to the fact that firstly it allows for longer resection period in absence of TUR syndrome and secondly simultaneous coagulation and resection provides better hemostasis.
- *Beneficial in cardiac patients on pacemaker*: In contrast to the monopolar technique, the energy used in bipolar does not pass through the patient's body and hence the energy is localized exclusively in the prostate, with limited negative effects at a distance. This is an advantage over monopolar, where current passing through the body of the patient can lead to possible malfunction of cardiac pacemaker.

## AUTHOR'S TECHNIQUE OF BIPOLAR TURP (ANATOMICAL TRANSURETHRAL RESECTION OF PROSTATE)

### Anatomical Basis

Prostate is mainly supplied by two branches of inferior vesical artery: (1) urethral and (2) capsular artery. In BPH, adenoma is mainly supplied by urethral arteries (Flocks, 1937). Prostatovesical junction is penetrated by urethral arteries posterolaterally, which approach bladder neck from 1 o'clock to 5 o'clock and 7 o'clock to 11 o'clock positions. Resection of median and lateral lobes is in accordance with blood supply of prostate, taking care of the bleeders at the capsular level and devascularizing the lobes. Resection can be completed rapidly with less bleeding. This is especially helpful in patients with larger glands and in high-risk patients.

Before starting TURP, cystoscopy should be performed in order to exclude any other pathology in the bladder and to establish the landmarks:
- Bladder neck
- Ureteric orifices
- Verumontanum
- Sphincter.

*Step 1: Resection of Median Lobe (Figs. 12.1 to 12.3)*

Median lobe is resected first. Resection is started at 5 o'clock position by creating a tough from bladder neck till verumontanum followed by a similar trough at 7 o'clock position. This causes devascularisation of median lobe and it is resected rapidly with less bleeding. This creates a channel for better irrigation.

*Step 2: Resection at 12 o'clock and Left Lobe (Figs. 12.4A and B)*

Lateral lobes are resected one after another. Resection is done at 12 o'clock position followed by a trough made at 1 o'clock position with plane of resection up to the capsule of prostate. Then lateral lobe is resected rapidly with less bleeding.

*Step 3: Resection of Right Lobe*

After that right lateral lobe is resected in similar fashion starting a trough creation at 11 o'clock position. Apical tissue and tissue next to verumontanum is resected Finally (Step 4). Shaving of small residual tissues over the capsule is the next step (Step 5). Hemostasis is the last part of the procedure (Step 6). [Figs. 12.5A to D (step 3 to 6)].

Author with experience of more than 40 years has performed B-TURP in glands more than 150 g, with this technique without a single incidence of blood transfusion and TUR syndrome.

## Bipolar Transurethral Resection of the Prostate

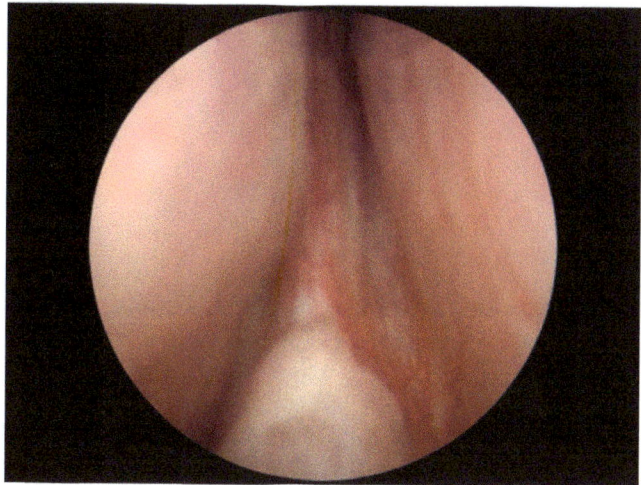

**Fig. 12.1:** Median lobe (endoscopic view).

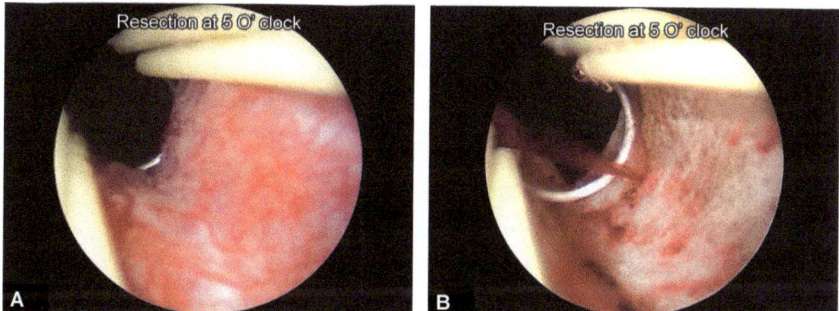

**Figs. 12.2A and B:** Resection at 5 o'clock position and coagulation of Budenoch artery.

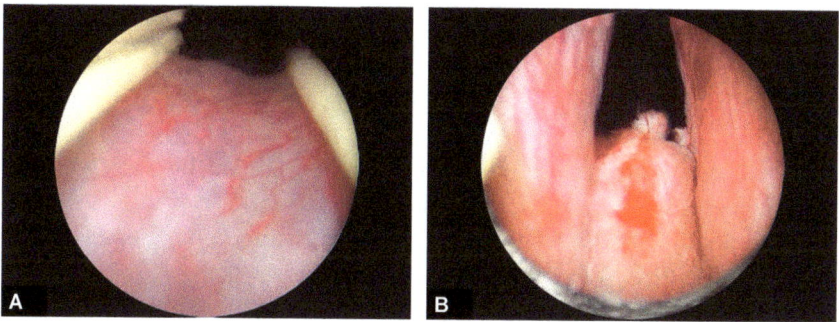

**Figs. 12.3A and B:** (A) Resection at 7 o'clock; and (B) Channel created after median lobe resection.

## Handbook of Transurethral Resection (TUR) Technique

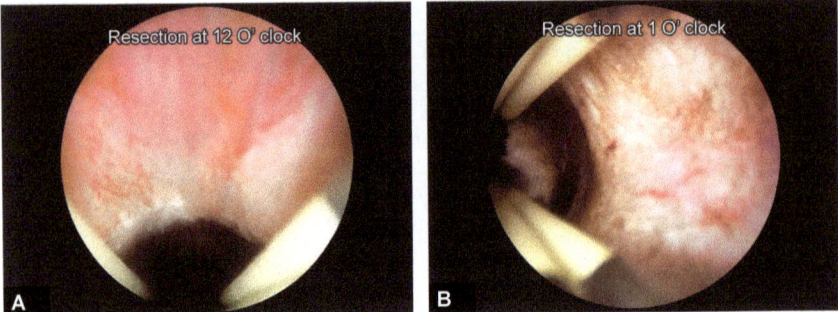

**Figs. 12.4A and B:** (A) Resection at 12 o'clock position; and (B) Trough creation up to capsule at 1 o'clock.

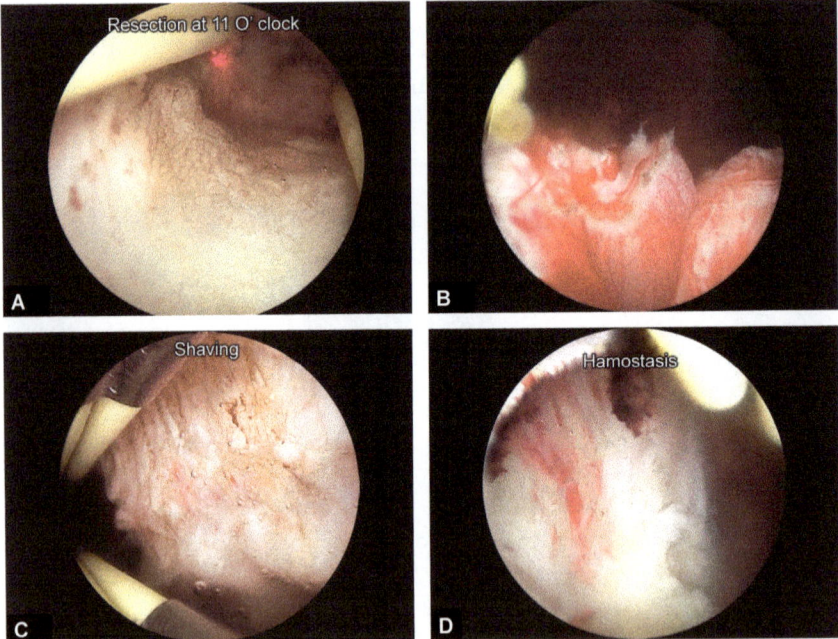

**Figs. 12.5A to D:** (A) Step 3: Resection of right lobe; and (B) Step 4: Apical tissue resection lateral to verumontanum; (C) Step5: Shaving; and (D) Step 6: Hemostasis.

## ▎TIPS AND TRICKS

- Resect one lobe after another—second lobe should be resected after complete resection and hemostasis of one lobe.
- Movement of the loop should be slow—to ensure better hemostasis in bipolar TURP.
- Landmarks should always be kept in mind while resecting.
- Perforation should be avoided during initial resection to avoid fluid absorption.

## RECOMMENDATIONS OF 2017 EAU GUIDELINES

According to EAU guidelines, bipolar- or monopolar-TURP should be offered to surgically treat patients of moderate-to-severe lower urinary tract symptoms (LUTS) in men with prostate size of 30–80 mL (Level of Evidence 1a, Grade of Recommendation A).

## CONCLUSION

Bipolar-TURP is an attractive alternative to M-TURP in patients with moderate-to-severe LUTS secondary to bladder outlet obstruction, as B-TURP has equal efficacy with a relatively low perioperative morbidity.

In RCTs with a follow-up of up to 5 years, safety and efficacy profile of B-TURP has been found to be comparable to M-TURP. Because of its safety profile, it is one of the reliable training techniques for urology residents.

## BIBLIOGRAPHY

1. Autorino R, Damiano R, Di Lorenzo G, et al. Four-year outcome of a prospective randomised trial comparing bipolar plasmakinetic and monopolar transurethral resection of the prostate. Eur Urol. 2009;55:922-9.
2. Burke N, Whelan JP, Goeree L, et al. Systematic review and meta-analysis of transurethral resection of the prostate versus minimally invasive procedures for the treatment of benign prostatic obstruction. Urology. 2010;75:1015-22.
3. Cornu JN, Ahyai S, Bachmann A, et al. A Systematic Review and Meta-analysis of Functional Outcomes and Complications Following Transurethral Procedures for Lower Urinary Tract Symptoms Resulting from Benign Prostatic Obstruction: An Update. Eur Urol. 2015;67:1066-96.
4. Issa MM. Technological advances in transurethral resection of the prostate: bipolar versus monopolar TURP. J Endourol. 2008;22:1587-95.
5. Miki M, Loritani N. TUR in Saline: TURis. Tokyo, Japan: Olympus Corporation Publishing; 2004.
6. Mamoulakis C, Sofras F, de la Rosette J, et al. Bipolar versus monopolar transurethral resection of the prostate for lower urinary tract symptoms secondary to benign prostatic obstruction. Cochrane Database Syst Rev. 2014;1:CD009629.
7. Omar MI, Lam TB, Alexander CE, et al. Systematic review and meta-analysis of the clinical effectiveness of bipolar compared with monopolar transurethral resection of the prostate (TURP). BJU Int. 2014;113:24-35.
8. Tefekli A, Muslumanoglu AY, Baykal M, et al. A hybrid technique using bipolar energy in transurethral prostate surgery: a prospective randomized comparison. J Urol. 2005;174:1339-43.

# Chapter 13

# Postoperative Care Following Transurethral Resection of the Prostate

*R Manikandan*

## INTRODUCTION

The postoperative care after transurethral procedures concerns the need for catheter (catheter care, irrigation, and traction), management of bleeding, electrolyte imbalances, and other complications.

## CATHETER INSERTION

The postoperative care starts immediately after the transurethral resection of the prostate (TURP) with catheter insertion. Urethral catheter is mandatory following TURP. In rare instances, after potassium titanyl phosphate (KTP) laser evaporation of prostate, urethral catheter is dispensed with.

The main reasons for catheterization are:
- To assess the presence and amount of hematuria
- To prevent clot retention (with irrigation)
- To provide tamponade effect (with or without traction)
- Decrease discomfort of voiding through injured ulcerated urethra.

### Difficult Catheterization

It is one of the common problems encountered following TURP. Even with adequate amount of lubricant and little force, the catheter does not enter the bladder. Most often the obstruction is at the level of bladder neck, especially in those with large median lobes. In these patients, the resection of the lobe results in a "gutter" in the prostate and a bladder neck "shelf" proximally. It also occurs with inadvertent subtrigonal perforation.

In such situations, a few methods can be tried. The first simple method is to do a rectal examination. The catheter tip position can be felt. It should be retracted a few centimeters, and with digital pressure, the prostate gutter can be flattened and catheter pushed into the bladder with finger. If Guyon's catheter introducer is available, it can be used. Since it is placed *within* the catheter, it is similar to insertion of urethral dilator. The other option is the use of Maryfield introducer. It is a sturdy instrument and may be traumatic if used without due care.

The other simple method is to introduce a guidewire using a cystoscope and threading the catheter over it.

## Irrigation

Though we usually ensure absolute hemostasis after TURP or transurethral resection of bladder tumor (TURBT), some small ooze may occur during recovery from anesthesia due to blood pressure fluctuations. Even introduction of catheter may abrade the fossa and start bleeding. Bleeding results in the formation of clots and ensuing catheter block. This may aggravate minimal bleeding in some instances. To prevent this, it is necessary to start the irrigation immediately and continue it. The irrigation speed should be such that the returns are light pink to clear. The clarity should be such as to be able to read paper print through the column of urine in the tube. If the color is darker, it is better to do a repeat cystoscopy and clear the bleeders. Though few centers do TURPs with no irrigation after the procedure, it is always better to have the irrigation in flow in the immediate postoperative period.

Irrigation can be a double edged sword too. If the patient is having catheter block and is on irrigation, he may go into painful retention rapidly due to fast bladder filling. Continuous drainage of urine through the catheter should be ensured at least every hour, to detect catheter block early.

Irrigation may be continued for 1 or 2 days, till the urine is light pink to clear even after stopping the irrigation for few minutes. If the patient has a catheter traction, it is better to continue irrigation for a few hours after releasing traction. Occasionally, there might be bleeding immediately after release of traction.

## Traction

Though postoperative irrigation is still practiced in almost all centers, many resectionist questioned the need for postoperative traction and place the catheter without traction.

Traction is necessary when the returns are not clear with irrigation and we suspect venous ooze or uncontrollable venous sinus bleed. The traction should be such as to gine a superoinferior compression to the prostate fossa. Presence of residual prostate lobes may not give adequate tamponade with this traction since adequate compression cannot be achieved.

The catheter balloon is inflated to 40–50 mL so that it does not migrate down even with the application of traction. Traction catheter can be fixed to the thighs or the abdomen. Thigh traction provides a relatively better compression of fossa than the abdomen fixation. In case of thigh traction, catheter can be stretched till mid or distal thigh near knee joint, depending on the severity of bleeding. In those with significant residual prostate, more traction is necessary.

In case of abdominal traction, the catheter is stretched and fixed to the lower abdomen below the umbilicus. This is more comfortable to the patients since he can move his lower limbs without restriction. But, the degree of compression is lesser.

*Salvaris traction*: In the instances, when thigh traction alone is insufficient, or there is pericatheter bleed, Salvaris traction can be given. An iodine-soaked gauze is wound around the catheter and compressed against the meatus. This gives better hemostasis with compression at both ends. The important point to note is that, since it causes high pressure at the level of meatus, prolonged application beyond 6-12 hours can cause pressure necrosis and later meatal stenosis.

In rare instances, with very large sinus openings, balloon needs to be inflated *within* the prostatic fossa. This should be accomplished with image intensifier guidance. The chances of sphincter damage are higher with this kind of traction.

The duration of traction should not be more than 24 hours other than in extreme circumstances. The safer option would be to release the traction by 12 hours if there is no significant bleeding. Prolonged traction will cause bladder neck ischemia and can result in bladder neck stenosis. Prolonged pressure on the sphincters may cause neuropraxia or neurotmesis and patient may develop incontinence.

## INVESTIGATIONS

If the blood loss is high in subjective assessment, hemoglobin and hematocrit may be assessed after 6 hours. In those patients with large glands (>50 g), prolonged operative duration (>90 min), excess bleeding or use of water as irrigant, serum sodium needs to be assessed postoperatively.

## Monitoring

Other than the routine postoperative monitoring, urine output should be monitored every 30-60 minutes to ensure clear color and continuous drainage to pick up catheter block early. Blood pressure should be well controlled to avoid opening up of cauterized venous sinuses. The patient resumes normal diet as soon as they recover from the anesthetic and ambulated as early as possible. Routine DVT prophylaxis is not necessary. In susceptible patients, TED stockings can be applied. Since retching and vomiting can increase the chances of bleed, antiemetics can be given to patients with nausea, especially after general anesthesia. For the patients who have undergone TURBT, vigorous catheter manipulation needs to be avoided. The catheter tip may impinge onto the raw surface of tumor bed and may initiate bleeding.

Straining during defecation may precipitate hematuria. Hence patients are advised to take stool softeners postoperatively for at least a week.

Bladder spasms may be precipitated after bladder neck resections and in those patients with short trigone. Anticholinergics will help in relieving the spasmodic pain. The inflated bulb will impinge on the rectum and the patient will have the urge to defecate. If the patient had evacuated the bowels or given enema on the day of surgery, the rectum will be empty and he just reassuring the patient is enough. Foley balloon bulb should be partially deflated to 10–15 mL while releasing the traction.

## ANALGESICS AND ANTIBIOTICS

Nonsteroidal anti-inflammatory drugs (NSAIDs) or synthetic opioids can be given for 2–3 days. Antibiotic usage is governed by the antibiotic policy of the institution. The antibiotic prophylaxis is usually continued for 4–5 days after the surgery. Some surgeons give cholinergic agonists (bethanechol) postoperatively for successful trial void. But it has just level 5 evidence for recommendation.

Catheter is usually removed after 72 hours. In some centers, it is removed after 48 hours. The main criteria is the presence of clear urine.

Patients are advised to avoid strenuous exertion for a minimum of 3 weeks. This reduces the chances for delayed bleeding and clot retention.

*Management of reactionary bleeding*: This usually occurs in postoperative period when patient has been shifted from operation room to the postoperative recovery room. This happens if some of the bleeders have reopened, or traction has become loose in cases where sinuses were opened.

## MANAGEMENT

- First check irrigation is going on properly with good return.
- Apply traction and observe for the color of the irrigant.
- Sometimes balloon slips into fossa and stretching capsule results in constant oozing. Deflate balloon, push the catheter in bladder, reinflate and give traction.
- If not controlled, shift the patient in operation theater, reinspect fossa and coagulate any bleeding spots.
- Further steps are same as primary hemorrhage, insert three-way Foley catheter. Inflate the balloon more than the size of the fossa and apply traction. Bleeding usually stops if bleeding only from venous sinuses and maintain it for 24 hours.

- If the bleeding is not decreasing in spite of waiting for sufficient time, it may be due to opening of deep sinuses.
- Deflate balloon and inflate only 5–10 cc and pull balloon in prostatic fossa, at sphincteric area and give a resistance. Inflate balloon in fossa as per approximate capacity and observe for bleeding. In majority of cases, the bleeding stops and after 24 hours balloon can be deflated, pushing into the bladder with or without traction.
- Additionally rectodigital compression can be applied to achieve tamponade.
- If all the above options fails to control bleeding, without wasting time open bladder to look for any bleeder and coagulate.
- Inspect fossa thoroughly and see for any obvious bleeder. If generalized oozing, pack the fossa with long bandage soaked in Betadine solution around Foleys catheter and bring one end of bandage out through the suprapubic wound. Close the bladder over a suprapubic catheter.
- Maintain it for 24–48 hours and if vitals are stable and bleeding under control, packing can be removed.
- Apart from the above management options following measures are to be adopted: intravenous fluids, blood transfusions, and antibiotics.
- Rule out any bleeding diathesis. Take history of aspirin or antiplatelets which may have been missed and treat accordingly.
- Rarely, transfemoral super selective angio-embolization may be required.

# Chapter 14

# Complications in Transurethral Resection of Prostate

*PVLN Murthy*

## INTRODUCTION

The safety and efficacy of transurethral resection of the prostate (TURP) has improved after the advent of glycine as an irrigant, improvised electrocautery generators, video TURP and bipolar transurethral resection (TUR).

Tables 14.1 to 14.3 enumerate the common complications and their incidence rates.

The complications can be broadly classified into intraoperative, early, and late postoperative complications.

## INTRAOPERATIVE COMPLICATIONS

*Problems of instrument introduction*: These cannot be called complications per se, but, they need rectification before proceeding with surgery.

**Table 14.1:** Enumeration of common complications.

| Type of complication | Early 1990 (%) | Recent 2015 (%) |
|---|---|---|
| Clot retention | 3.3 | 5 |
| Bleeding and transfusion | 6.4 | 2 |
| Transurethral resection of the prostate (TURP) syndrome | 2 | 0 |
| Capsular perforation | 0.9 | 4 |
| Hydronephrosis | 0.3 | 0 |
| Epididymitis/urinary tract infection (UTI) | 3.9 | 4 |
| Urosepsis | 0.2 | 0 |
| Failure to void | 6.5 | 5 |
| Incontinence | 0.3–30 | 1.0 |

**Table 14.2:** Enumeration of incidence rates.

| Others | Incidence (%) |
|---|---|
| Bladder neck contracture | 6 |
| Stricture urethra | 4 |
| Delayed hemorrhage | 2 |
| Sexual dysfunction | 3 |

**Table 14.3:** Associated morbidity: early and recent.

| Associated morbidity | Early | Recent |
|---|---|---|
| Cardiac arrhythmias | 1.1 | Not available |
| Myocardial infarction | 0.05 | 0 |
| Pulmonary embolism | NA | 0 |
| Pneumonia | NA | 0 |
| Chronic obstructive pulmonary disease (COPD) | 0.5 | NA |
| Deep vein thrombosis (DVT) | NA | 0 |
| Mortality | 0.23 | 0 |

*Phimosis*: This is not uncommon in this part of the world. Most often it is noted during clinical examination or on the table. Circumcision (prior consent mandatory) or limited dorsal slit suffices to allow instrument introduction. If circumcision is planned, it is advisable to complete the procedure including suturing, prior to starting resection. In case of poor hemostasis at the end needing immediate traction, completing the suturing with catheter under traction will be difficult.

*Meatal calibration*: Dorsal meatotomy can be performed with Sachse's meatotome or Otis urethrotome to facilitate the introduction of the resectoscope. Ventral meatotomy with a scalpel, using a metal sound in the urethra as a guide can also be done. Calibration with metal sounds up to 28 F is routinely practiced by many urologists to facilitate smooth passage of 26 F resectoscope.

*Urethral calibration*: Most urologists calibrate the urethra with metal sounds till 28 Fr prior to introduction of resectoscope. Blind internal urethrotomy with Otis urethrotome or visual internal urethrotomy using urethrotome and Sachse's knife is also an option. The free movement of the resectoscope within the urethra is essential to prevent later complications like stricture urethra. In situations where the resectoscope is snuggly fitting and excursion of the sheath is difficult, the inner 24 F sheath can be used and a suprapubic trocar (Reuter suprapubic trocar) provides continuous outflow especially in large glands. In those with narrow penile urethra and comparatively patulous bulbar urethra, perineal urethrotomy can be done. Procedure is completed through the urethrotomy and the urethral opening closed at the end of the procedure.

*Intraoperative priapism (4%)*: It is not uncommon for a patient to develop priapism during TURP or even before the introduction of the sheath. It may occur with any mode of anesthesia and often persists stubbornly despite all therapeutic measures. Treatment is usually with intracavernosal phenylephrine injections. One milliliter of phenylephrine (10 mg/mL) is diluted in 49 mL of normal saline (0.2 mg/mL) and 1–2 mL injected every 10–15 min. intracavernosally till detumescence occurs. Other commonly used drugs are intravenous ketamine, glycopyrrolate, and terbutaline. If detumescence does not occur, it is safe to abandon the procedure. The other option in such patients is to do a perineal urethrotomy and complete the procedure.

*Hypothermia*: Room-temperature irrigation can cause substantial decrease in core body temperatures especially in continuous flow resection. Other factors that can contribute to hypothermia are larger glands, longer resection times, small body habitus, low body weight and lower room temperature and elderly patients. Hypothermia can cause cardiac stress, bradycardia, decreased cardiac output, increased mean arterial pressure, and peripheral vascular resistance. Apnea, angina, and myocardial infarction (MI) have been reported at temperatures around 35°C. Use of body warmers, adequate covering with blankets and warming the irrigant to body temperature will help to combat hypothermia.

## Bleeding

Bleeding during the resection procedure is a norm rather than exception. The amount of bleeding and blood loss alone makes the difference. The amount of intraoperative bleeding varies depending upon factors like prostate size, resection time, and technique of resection and experience of the surgeon. The rate of bleeding can be assessed and can be termed "alarming", if there is fresh blood trickling through the scope at the time of emptying the bladder/dark red effluent/red vision in the scope.

Knowledge of the vascular anatomy of the prostate, as described by Flock is useful. The main arterial supply is between the 5 o'clock and 7 o'clock position and 11 o'clock and 1 o'clock positions. If the bleeder directly spurts on to the scope, withdrawing the sheath into the urethra might show the bleeder. Meticulous inspection of the resected areas helps in identifying the bleeder. If the vision is too poor to see anything, the height of the irrigant may be increased for a short duration. This is particularly helpful in venous bleed.

Identifying the bleeders is half job done. Application of coagulation current directly to the spurter is useful in small bleeders. In case of broad venous bleeders, applying the current over the feeding vessel and broad based coagulation will be fruitful.

In those patient in whom nothing works, broad lumen catheter is inserted into the bladder and balloon is filled to 50-60 mL. Traction is applied and bladder is irrigated. If the bleeding is not controlled with this maneuver, under fluoroscopy guidance, catheter balloon can be inflated directly within the prostate cavity. Else, the final option is completing the procedure by open prostatectomy and packing the fossa.

Preoperative evaluation of patient's coagulation profile and stoppage of blood thinners are essential to prevent excessive bleeding. We must ensure that the blood pressure is normal at the time of hemostasis at the end of the procedure so that significant bleeding points are not masked by hypotension.

Intraoperative bleeding may be more significant in cases of infection and resection immediately after acute urinary retention because of congested gland. Administration of antiandrogens like finasteride or dutasteride for a period of 2-4 weeks reduces intraoperative bleeding.

Transfusion rates should be less than 1% (0.4-7.1%). Careful fulguration of arterial bleeders by point coagulation decreases the chance of delayed hemorrhage that can result from the sloughing of tissue secondary to massive fulguration of the prostatic fossa.

Capsular perforation or opening of venous sinusoidal plexus results in darkish blue venous bleeding. It is not absolute necessity to terminate resection when venous sinuses are opened, but the chances of fluid intravasation should be borne in mind and the procedure should be completed as fast as possible. Sinus bleeding responds to catheter traction and irrigation. Catheter block should be avoided; otherwise this results in bladder/prostatic fossa distension causing further bleeding.

## Perforation

*Extravasation of fluid (capsular perforation)*: It is not uncommon to have small, insignificant perforations of the bladder neck/prostatic capsule. If a major perforation occurs during the initial part of the resection, large amounts of fluid may extravasate into the retroperitoneum causing discomfort and exacerbation of TUR syndrome. Patients under spinal anesthesia immediately complain of suprapubic pain/discomfort due to peritoneal irritation. If there is suprapubic fullness, it is better to put a drain in the space of Retzius and abandon the procedure, only to take up after 48 hours. The resection can be continued in case of small perforations.

Another sign of significant perforation/extravasation is distortion of prostatic urethra in which the lumen is narrowed and the length of the prostatic urethra is lengthened. The bladder neck and trigone may appear distant. Perforations posteriorly in the prostatic capsule usually occur at the bladder neck area. If the perforations are in this position or prostatic urethra is distorted, cystogram should be performed. Cystogram is also indicated if there is abdominal discomfort or abdominal distension. In the event of intraperitoneal perforation of bladder, one has to explore and close the perforation. Anterior and lateral perforations occasionally occur and can be managed with catheter drainage if there is minimal extravasation, otherwise they need drainage. Careful monitoring of electrolytes is essential in first 24-hours postoperative.

In rare instances, it may not be recognized intraoperatively and the patient may develop abdominal distension in the recovery room. If the distension is minimal, a drain can be placed under local anesthesia and observed. The telltale sign of the bladder perforation or gross prostate capsule perforation is the absence of complete returns on bladder wash with Tommey syringe or Ellick's evacuator. Persistant increase in abdominal distension is an indication for laparotomy. Though some intraperitoneal fluid seepage may be present, gross ascites suggests possibility of intraperitoneal perforation and associated inadvertent bowel injury needs to be ruled out. Even with extraperitoneal injuries, when associated with gross extravasations, exploration and repair of the rent will reduce the drain output and helps in faster healing.

## TURP SYNDROME

It occurs as a consequence of absorption into prostatic venous sinuses of fluids used to irrigate the bladder during the operation. It happens when a venous sinus is opened or capsular perforation occurs early in the resection or when resection time is prolonged. Symptoms and signs are varied and unpredictable, and result from fluid overload and electrolyte imbalance like hyponatremia.

The syndrome is characterized by confusion, hypertension, bradycardia, nausea, vomiting, and visual disturbances. Dilutional hyponatremia is the cause and symptoms usually do not manifest until the serum sodium drops to less than 125 mEq. Hypertension and mental confusion are the predominant symptoms. Hypotension, bradycardia or restlessness secondary to hyponatremia may follow. The CNS changes such as visual disturbances, disorientation, stupor, coma and seizures have been attributed to hyponatremia (any irrigating fluid), hypoglycemia and hyperammonemia (with glycine). Diminished vision extending to blindness has been reported. The onset may occur any time 30 minutes after start of surgery up to 6 hours, after surgery is completed. Vision usually returns to normal 2-12 hours after surgery. Cardiovascular symptoms like increased CVP, bradycardia, hypertension, cardiovascular collapse, and ECG changes occur due to intravascular absorption of fluid.

In monopolar TURP, sterile water or glycine is the medium of irrigation which are associated with electrolyte imbalance or CNS toxicity apart from associated morbidity with fluid overload. In case of bipolar TURP where saline is the irrigant, the risk of electrolyte imbalance may not be there, but cardiopulmonary failure can occur when large volume of fluid is absorbed.

These symptoms are recognized at the earliest in those under spinal anesthesia. If a perforation occurs or venous sinuses are opened during resection, a loop diuretic like furosemide 40-120 mg should be administered intravenously and normal saline infusion to be continued. In patients with severe hyponatremia, 3% hypertonic saline may be necessary and infused depending on the sodium deficit. Resection time should be limited to 60-90 minutes and water column around 70 cm height to be kept to prevent TURP syndrome. It is safe to give loop diuretic routinely during the final phases of resection as we approach the capsule.

## Undermining the Trigone

This complication was more in earlier days, when Schmidt's visual obturator was not used. On blind insertion of the sheath with large median lobe, the scope undermines the trigone and lifts up the median lobe. Nowadays, it happens due to overzealous resection of bladder neck and proximal prostatic urethra in the floor. The prostatic fossa forms a gutter, going beneath the trigone. In this situation it is better to pass a Foley catheter over a guidewire at the end of the resection. Otherwise, the catheter tip can produce false passage under the trigone and inflated balloon will further worsens resulting in bladder neck—prostatic urethral dissociation.

*Resection of ureteral orifice*: Resection of ureter or ureteral orifice (UO) inadvertently or by carelessness can occur while resecting the intravesical projection (median lobe) of prostate. It is mandatory to visualize the UO in such configurations before resection. If the UOs are too close to resection, pure cutting current setting should be employed to minimize the damage. If a coagulating current was used during the resection of UOs, stenting of ureter should be done and stents are left for 4-6 weeks. Postoperative ultrasound scanning should be done to evaluate for any ureteral stricture. Preprocedural CPE will help to understand the configuration of the gland and landmarks of resection as well.

## EARLY COMPLICATIONS

*Clot retention*: This requires through evacuation of clots not only from the bladder, but prostatic fossa as well. Adherent clots should be resected from the prostatic fossa to unearth the bleeders. Systematic examination of prostatic fossa for bleeding sites should be conducted using the irrigation fluid under low pressure. A common area in which undetected postoperative hemorrhage occurs is the anterior bladder neck where pieces of prostatic tissue often pulled in during resection and reside in side the bladder neck. Careful observation of this area is essential if there is no obvious bleeding points are not found on re-exploration.

Rarely, open surgical exploration may be necessary, for direct fulguration or ligation of bleeding points. Vesicocapsulotomy may be useful in this situation to directly see and ligate the vessels. A circumferential bladder neck suture may be of benefit in resistant cases and rarely should it be necessary to pack the prostatic fossa. Placement of a Foley balloon catheter (24 F) with in prostatic fossa is advocated in troublesome cases.

If troublesome postoperative bleeding continues, one should suspect primary fibrinolysis and intravascular coagulation especially in patients with adenocarcinoma of prostate and seek the help of hematologist.

*Urinary incontinence*: Urinary incontinence following TURP is a rare complication and an etiology can be multifactorial. While early incontinence may occur in up to 30–40% of patients, persistant late incontinence occurs in less than 1% of cases. The degree of incontinence can range from urgency with urge incontinence to stress incontinence to continuous incontinence. Patient factors, disease factors, and surgical factors may contribute to post-prostatectomy incontinence (PPI).

The patient factors include obesity, frail elderly patients, those with associated neurological conditions, primary detrusor over activity, etc. Old frail patients and those with neurological disorders may have inherent weakness of the sphincter mechanism, leading to incontinence. These patients usually have urge incontinence or minimal stress incontinence. Some patients have idiopathic detrusor over activity. They have urgency with urge incontinence and usually respond to anticholinergics.

Benign prostatic hyperplasia (BPH) disease per se can cause functional modification in the detrusor myofascial contraction mechanism of the detrusor resulting in urgency and urge incontinence. Among those with features of detrusor overactivity prior to TURP, 30% respond well and storage symptoms including urgency and urge incontinence settles with TURP. In the rest, some amount of urgency and urge incontinence may persist. Poor bladder compliance due to detrusor wall thickening may also contribute in some cases. Anticholinergics help in these groups of patients too.

The surgical factors also contribute to PPI. Damage to the external urethral sphincter and resultant continuous vertical incontinence is an urologist's nightmare. Some amount of neuropraxia and incontinence in the early postoperative period can be expected after resection of large prostates.

But, the incontinence is usually urge incontinence or minimal stress leak. It settles with time, in addition to Kegel's exercises and anticholinergics. Gross vertical incontinence is most likely caused by extensive resection of the sphincter. Great care should be taken while resecting the gland around the verumontanum. Extensive resection beyond verumontanum should be avoided. The sphincter is horse shoe shaped, with the bulky part situated anteriorly. So, extensive use of diathermy in the anterior aspect close to the verumontanum, should be avoided.

The other cause for incontinence is persistence of small part of apical tissue after TURP. This prevents close apposition of the sphincter and may lead to incontinence.

Post-prostatectomy incontinence may be a temporary impairment, which may spontaneously resolve. Most patients recover urinary continence within the first 6–12 months following surgery. Early incontinence is usually related to urge incontinence, either because of storage symptoms due to the prostatic fossa healing and associated urinary tract infection or detrusor overactivity and decreased compliance caused by long-standing bladder outflow obstruction by BPH.

The first step in management of PPI is observation with anticholinergics and Kegel's exercises. If there is no improvement, urodynamic study with cystoscopy is indicated. Bladder contractility, compliance, overactivity and the presence of residual apical lobe can be assessed. Treatment can be initiated depending on the findings. The integrity of the sphincter can be assessed by hydrostatic test during cystoscopy. Scope is placed just distal to the sphincter and the irrigant flow is stopped and restarted alternately. Hydrostatic pressure of the irrigant stimulated sphincter contraction, which can be seen. Absence of this reflux increases the suspicion of sphincteric injury.

The management of PPI has changed and improved significantly after the advent of male urethral slings and artificial urinary sphincter. Management of sphincter injury depends on the severity. Minimal stress leak can be managed by conservative management. Bulbourethral slings can be used in those with moderate leak. Artificial urinary sphincter is preferred in cases of detrusor underactivity and moderate incontinence.

## Urinary Retention

Underactive detrusor and incomplete resection are attributed to postoperative retention following TURP. Patients at increased risk of having weak streams or inability to void spontaneously postoperatively, such as patients with poorly controlled DM, chronic urinary retention, and neurogenic cause of retention, need detailed evaluation by UDS before taking up for TURP. Benefit of doubt of resection to be given for carefully selected group of patients as they void better after TURP. Patients who void incompletely leaving behind large amount of residual urine improve on CIC over a period of time. A reevaluation of bladder neck for residual gland by cystoscopy is mandatory before putting the patient on conservative management.

*Infection (3.5–21.6%)*: Urine should be sterile before TURP and parental antibiotic to be continued for 24–48 hours postoperatively. In men with postoperative urinary tract infection (UTI), postoperative oral urinary antiseptics to be continued for 2 weeks as the fossa is raw. Rarely, these patients can develop febrile UTI/pyelonephritis or septic shock (2.3%), especially who are on long-term catheters. TURP can produce VUR due to tampering of trigone/VUJ and infected urine can cause PN. Postoperative pyuria is expected and do not indicate UTI all the time. Administration of antibiotics should not be given without urine culture report.

## LATE COMPLICATIONS

### Urethral Stricture

It occurs in less than 5% of patients following TURP. Many randomized clinical trials reported the rates of bladder neck contracture and stricture urethra were 4.7% and 3.8% respectively (Lee et al.). The site of stricture can be meatal/submeatal (navicular fossa), proximal bulbar or penoscrotal. The basic determining factors for the development of stricture include, prostate volume/resection time, surgeon's experience, catheter size (>20 F), mismatch between resectoscope size and urethral caliber and presence of prostate cancer. Routine calibration of urethra by metal sounds 2 F more than the resectoscope size, meatotomy or urethrotomy by Otis urethrotome reduce the incidence significantly. It is observed that the incidence of stricture is equally associated with monopolar or bipolar TURP and PVP. Majority of strictures respond to either periodic dilatation or optical urethrotomy and rarely require urethroplasty. The old teaching of routine calibration by a 24 F metal boogie, 8 weeks postoperative breaks the bladder neck synechiae or allow a stricture to be detected before it becomes severe enough to cause management problem. One should be careful while managing membranous urethral stenosis/stricture where dilatation alone needs to be done rather than optical urethrotomy to prevent sphincter damage.

### Bladder Neck Contracture

Bladder neck contracture (BNC) is not an uncommon complication after TURP and the exact cause is not known. However, some predisposing causes have been identified. They are excessive use of coagulating current during resection, small fibrous glands, prolonged and excessive catheter traction to control bleeding and over resection. Bladder neck incisions and leaving a strip of mucosa at 12 o'clock have been practiced to reduce the incidence by half (Lee et al.).

Bladder neck contracture responds to cold cut or laser at 6 o'clock or 12 o'clock positions or Mercedes Benz incision when there is a concentric stenosis. Electroresection should be avoided as induces further fibrosis. In intractable cases open bladder neck V-Y plasty has been advocated.

*Sexual function*: Some men (30%) experience sexual dysfunction after TURP and complete recovery may take up to 1 year. The most common, long-term side effect of prostate surgery is retrograde ejaculation (dry climax, 48%).

Transurethral resection of the prostate causes retrograde ejaculation, which is a bothersome feature in some men, but its effect on erectile function is controversial. Long-term data suggests that TURP does not affect sexual function and indicate that erection problems precede TURP in this group of patients. In fact some patients claim that their sexual function improved after TURP probably due to resolution of lower urinary tract symptoms. Prospective studies measured by self-assessment questioners confirmed that TURP has no adverse effect on erectile function. Associated comorbidities like diabetes, hypertension and coronary heart disease contribute to erectile dysfunction in this group of patients.

## CONCLUSION

Transurethral resection of the prostate is a safe endoscopic operation. Similar to any other surgical procedure; TURP can result in various complications. Meticulous planning of the procedure, proper selection of patients, adequate counseling of patients and precise technique taking care of the nuances help in decreasing the incidence of complications.

## BIBLIOGRAPHY

1. Colau A, Lucet JC, Rufat P, et al. Incidence and risk factors of bacteriuria after transurethral resection of the prostate. Eur Urol. 2001;39:272-6.
2. Djavan B, Madersbacher S, Klingler C, et al. Urodynamic assessment of patients with acute urinary retention: is treatment failure after prostectomy predictable? J Urol. 1997;158:1829-33.
3. Geavlete B, Georgescu D, Multescu R, et al. Bipolar plasma vaporization vs monopoloar and bipolar TURP-A prospective randomized, long-term comparison. Urology. 2011;78:930-5.
4. Lee YH, Chiu AW, Huang JK. Comprehensive study of bladder neck contracture after transurethral resection of prostate. Urology. 2005;65:498-503.
5. Mariano RE. Irrigating solutions and TURP syndrome, section VII, Anesthesia for surgical subspecialities, In: Barash P (Ed). Clinical Anesthesia, 7th edition. Philadelphia, PA: Lippincott Williams and Wilkins; 2013.

6. Mitchell H. Sokoloff, Michel Kiarash. Complications of transurethral resection of the prostate. In: Taneja SS (Ed). Complications of Urologic Surgery: Prevention and Management, 4th edition. Philadelphia: Saunders Elsevier. 2009. pp. 279-94.
7. Muntener M, Aellig S, Kuettel R, et al. Sexual function after transurethral resection of the prostate (TURP): results of an independent prospective multicentre assessment of outcome. Eur Urol. 2007;52:510-6.
8. Pavone C, Abbadessa D, Scaduto G, et al. Sexual dysfunctions after transurethral resection of the prostate (TURP): evidence from a retrospective study on 264 patients. Arch Ital Urol Androl. 2015;87:8-13.
9. Puppo P, Bertolotto F, Introini C, et al. Bipolar transurethral resection in saline (TURis): outcome and complication rates after the first 1000 cases. J Endourol. 2009;23:1145-9.
10. Rassweiler J, Teber D, Kuntz R, et al. Complications of transurethral resection of the prostate (TURP)—incidence, management and prevention. Eur Urol. 2006;50:969-79.
11. Shantha TR. Intraoperative management of penile erection by using terbutaline. Anesthesiology. 1989;70:707-9.
12. Singh R, Asthana V, Sharma JP, et al. Effect of irrigation fluid temperature on core temperature and hemodynamic changes in transurethral resection of prostate under spinal anesthesia. Anesth Essays Res. 2014;8:209-15.
13. Söğütdelen E, Haberal HB, Fuad Guliyev F, et al. Urethral Stricture is an Unpleasant Complication after Prostate Surgery: A Critical Review of Current Literature. J Urol Surg. 2016;1:1-6.

# Index

*Page numbers followed by f refer to figure and t refer to table.*

## A

Abdominal traction  124
ACMI hemielectrode  86, 87*f*
Adenoma
    enucleation of  76
    lifting of  99*f*
    mucosa junction  73*f*, 74*f*
    separation of  79*f*
    yellowish brown appearance of  45*f*
Alexander's syringe  47
Amino acid, nonessential  64
Analgesics  125
Anesthesia  113
    epidural  27, 113
    general  30, 59, 113
    regional  27, 59
    spinal  27, 29, 113
Anesthetic management  29
Anticoagulants  28, 28*t*
Antiplatelets  28*t*
Apical lobe dissection  97
Avascular enucleated adenoma, resection of  81*f*

## B

Baumrucker system  4
Beta blockers  28
Bilobar gland  75
Bipolar circuit  14*f*
Bipolar energy  110
Bipolar enucleation, instruments for  68*f*
Bipolar resection  6
Bladder
    carcinoma  102
    distension  109
    diverticulum, tumor in  109
    dome, resection at  108
    endoscopic anatomy of  18
    irrigation, continuous  103
    jackstone calculus, large  52*f*
    lateral wall of  109*f*
    mucosa  24
    neck  23, 103, 118
        aperture  23*f*
        contracture  135
        elevation, severe  23*f*
        incision  53, 54*f*
        level of  99*f*
        proximal level of  79*f*
        shelf like elevation of  24*f*

perforation  111
    minimal  112*f*
tumor  111
    large  105*f*
    management  111
    wall, tumor on anterior  108
Bleeding  129
    and coagulopathy  32
    and transfusion  127
    control of  42
    postoperative  111
Blind obturator  11
Blood
    pressure  62
    transfusion rates, lower  117
Boat (canoe) shaped chips  40*f*
Bradycardia  131
Budenoch artery, coagulation of  119*f*
Bulbar urethra  19, 20*f*, 50
Button electrode  86

## C

Capsular fibers  96
Capsular perforation  127, 130
    with fat exposed  47*f*
Capsular resection, deeper  46*f*
Capsule, superficial layer of  46*f*
Carcinoma in situ, diffuse  106
Cardiac pacemaker  117
Cardiac rhythm either  12
Cardiovascular system assessment  28
Catheter insertion  122
Catheterization, difficult  122
    irrigation  123
    traction  123
Cautery artifact, reducing  110
Cerebral edema  65
Clot retention  127, 132
Collin's knife  107
    incision  9
Commissure incision, anterior  98*f*
Crisscrossing fibers  45
Cystoscope  7, 59
    sheath  7
Cystoscopy
    basic  39
    initial  104
    steps of  95
    white light  104
Cytal  65

## D

Deflate balloon  126
Diabetes mellitus  27
Diathermy
    and lasers  12
    cable  5
    equipment  5
    pads  36
Diode lasers  16
Distal sphincter  51$f$
Drainage hose  6
Drug intake  27
Dysuria  113

## E

Electric desiccation  106
Electrode  9
    design  85
Ellick's evacuator  9, 11, 47, 100
    classical  48$f$
    modified  47$f$
Endoscopes  3
    steam sterilization of  7
Endoscopic enucleation  67
Endoscopic surgery  3, 63
Energy shock waves, high  114
Enucleate small glands  82
Enucleation  82
    anatomical landmarks for  73
Epididymitis  127
Epidural analgesia  30
Equipment  94
Evacuator  5

## F

Fasting guidelines  29
Fine parallel fibers  46$f$
Finger-operated working element  8
Fluid, extravasation of  130
Fluorescence cystoscopy  104
Fresh frozen plasma  28

## G

Gas sterilization  7
Gland
    and capsule, differentiation of  44
    small wedges of  88
Glucose  65
Glycine  63, 64
    toxicity  31
Grooved rollerbar  85
Guyon's catheter  122

## H

Haemorrhage, primary  125
Hematuria  102
    painless  102
Hemoglobinuria, postoperative  63
Hemostasis  99
Holmium laser  17
    application for prostate  94
    enucleation of prostate  94
Holmium:yttrium-aluminum-garnet laser  94
Hydronephrosis  127
Hypertension, secondary to  27
Hyponatremia  131
Hypotension  131
Hypothermia  32, 129

## I

Incontinence  127
Infection  113
Insulin  28
Intensity focused ultrasound, high  114
International Prostate Symptom Score  83
Intracranial tumors, removal of  50
Intraoperative priapism  129
Intraperitoneal extravasation  112
Irrigants  31$t$
Irrigating solutions  104
Irrigation fluids  64
Irrigation tubes  5

## K

Karl Storz for bipolar enucleation of
            prostate  70$f$
Kegel's exercises  134
KTP lasers  17
KTP:YAG laser  16

## L

Laparoscopic surgery  18
Laser  15
    enucleation  94
    fibers  16
    types of  110
Lateral lobe dissection  97
Linear blood vessels  20$f$
Lithotomy position, classical  35
Litter's glands  19$f$
Lobe
    enucleation
        of lateral  97$f$
        of left lateral  91$f$
        of median  90$f$, 95, 95$f$, 96$f$

# Index

of right 77*f*
of right lateral 91*f*
from roof, separation of lateral 98
part of 97*f*
resection
    of left lateral 57*f*
    of median 118
    of right 118
small median 51*f*
Local microwave thermotherapy 114
Loop
    electrode 9
    for resection 5
    types of 5

## M

Mannitol 65
Meatal calibration 128
Meatus 18
Median lobe 119
    resection 119*f*
Membranous urethra 19
Mercier's bar 26
Minimally invasive surgery, advantages of 83
Mitomycin C, postoperative 111
Monopolar circuit 14*f*
Monopolar resection, cornerstone of 49
Morcellation 100
Mushroom button electrode from olympus 71*f*
Myocardial infarction 129

## N

Navicular fossa 18, 135
Nd:YAG laser 16, 17
Nesbit system 4
Nesbit technique 61
Nonmuscle invasive tumors 102
Nonsteroidal anti-inflammatory drugs 28, 125

## O

O'connor drape 62*f*
Obstructive pulmonary disease, chronic 27
Obstructive uropathy 27
Obturator 4
    externus 33
    nerve block 33
Occlusive lateral lobe 51*f*
Operation theater 3, 37
    set up 38*f*
Oral hypoglycemic agent 28
Ortho-phthalaldehyde 7
Otis urethrotome 59
Oxyhemoglobin 15

## P

Papillary low-grade tumors 110
Pearly white glistening capsule 45*f*
Penile urethra 19, 20*f*
Perforation 130
Peroneal nerve injury 35
Phimosis 128
Plasma
    button vaporization 89*f*
    energy, advantages of 86
    vaporization with button electrode 88
Plasmakinetic
    enucleation 67
    resection 14, 88
    vaporesection 91
    vaporization 84, 86
Plexiform blood vessels 20*f*
Prevent obturator jerk 109*f*
Proctoclysis enema 35
Prostate 62, 118
    ablation 2
    bipolar enucleation of 67
    chip being resected from 41*f*
    chips of exposed loop length 43
    fossa 123, 124, 132
    gland lateral lobes 23*f*
    groove
        in floor of 76*f*
        on roof of 76*f*
    parenchyma 41*f*, 42*f*
    resection of 50, 67
    surgery, history of 115
    vaporization of 94
Prostatectomy, open 67
Prostatic calcification 46*f*
Prostatic chips 47
Prostatic hyperplasia
    benign 2, 27, 54, 133
    management of benign 67
Prostatic obstruction 49
Prostatic tissue 55, 88
    bipolar resection of 116
    removal 116
Prostatic urethra 20, 21
Prostatovesical junction 118

## R

Reactionary bleeding, management of 125
Resected chips, removal of 47
Resection instruments 3
Resection near apex 61
Resectoscope
    inner sheath of 10
    outer sheath of 10
    sheath 4, 7

Respiratory system  29
Reuter suprapubic trocar  128
Robotic surgery  18
Roller electrode  85*f*
Rollerball  85
    electrode  9

## S

Sachse's knife  128
Saline, normal  65
Salvaris traction  124
Schmidt's obturator  4, 39
Schmidt's visual obturator  132
Sexual function  136
Sorbitol  65
Sphincter  118
Spinal anesthesia, contraindications for  30
Squamous cell carcinomas  102
Sterile water  64
Sterilization  6
Stern-McCarthy resectoscope  50

## T

Toomey's evacuators  100
Toomey's syringe  9, 47, 48, 48*f*
Transurethral catheter  110
Transurethral enucleation  67
    of prostate  68, 83
        with bipolar  67, 69*f*, 71*f*, 72*f*
    resection of prostate  67
Transurethral incision  50, 61
    of prostate  50, 53, 54*f*
Transurethral monopolar resection of prostate  49
Transurethral procedures  1
Transurethral prostatectomy  49
Transurethral resection  2, 3, 34, 40, 60, 136
    basics of  39
    complications of  111
    instruments for  37*f*
    of bladder tumor  27, 32, 102, 103, 104
        procedure  103
        surgery  32
    of prostate  2, 50, 55, 63, 67, 72*f*, 94, 115, 122
        anatomical  118
        anesthesia for  27
        author's technique of bipolar  118
        bipolar  115, 116
        complications of  31, 127
        efficacy of  127
        mechanism of bipolar  115
        monopolar  116
        safety of  127
        syndrome  31, 127, 131
        syndrome, treatment of  32
        technique of  58
        training in  60
    reaction  63
    syndrome  57, 63, 112, 118, 130
        elimination of  117
    technique of  39
Transurethral
    surgery, theater setup for  37
    vaporization of prostate  84, 91
Tumor at dome  108
Tumor location  107

## U

Urea  65
Ureteral orifice  26, 107
    resection of  132
    tumor involving  107
Ureteric catheter in situ  108*f*
Ureteric orifice  108*f*, 118
Urethra  103
    anatomy of  18
    dilated part of  18
    endoscopic anatomy of  18
    narrowed  53*f*
Urethral
    bougies  59
    calibration  128
    dilator, insertion of  122
    meatus, external  18
    sphincter, external  19, 21*f*
    stricture  135
Urethrotomy  50
Urinary
    incontinence  133
    retention  113, 134
    tract
        infection  127, 135
        symptoms, lower  121
Uroendoscopy, history of  1
Urological diseases, management of  1
Urosepsis  127
Urothelial cancer  102

## V

Vapor tome  86
Vaporcut electrode  85*f*
Vaporesection  88
Vaporization, concept of  84
Verumontanum  20, 118
Vessels, types of  100
Visual obturator  11

# Explore Health Science with Jaypeedigital

Portable
Searchable
Downloadable

## Main Features

- Unlimited concurrent users; no limitation on web reading
- Chapter-wise eBooks fully downloadable and printable
- Federated search within the platform
- Online medical dictionary
- Multilingual user interface
- Personalized features such as bookmark, favourites, previous test result and notes
- Available through yearly subscription

### eBooks
800+ Textbooks
2300+ Professional & Reference books

### Videos
4000+ Videos on live surgeries

### MCQs
70,000+ MCQs | 14 Specialities

# Jaypeedigital.com

an integrated online platform for eBooks, videos, MCQs and eJournals catering to the needs of students and professionals in health science

Join us on  www.facebook.com/JAYPEEDIGITAL    Follow us on  twitter.com/JAYPEEDIGITAL

Follow us on  : Jaypee Digital

EU GSPR Authorised Reprsentative
Logos Europe, 9 rue Nicolas Poussin
1700, La Rochelle, France
Phone: +33 (0) 6 67 93 73 78
E-mail: contact@logoseurope.eu

www.ingramcontent.com/pod-product-compliance
Ingram Content Group UK Ltd.
Pitfield, Milton Keynes, MK11 3LW, UK
UKHW050243150426
5217IPUK00005B/116